# DEFEATING
# the Big C

## the Martial Artist Way-with Diet and Discipline

MASTER ROY DAY

ISBN: 978-1-6847-0477-4 (sc)
ISBN: 978-1-6847-0476-7 (e)

Library of Congress Control Number: 2019906253

Cover Illustration by Master Roy Day

Lulu Publishing Services rev. date: 09/10/2019

# CONTENTS

Preface ................................................................................ xi

Chapter 1  The Diagnosis and the Fight ............................... 1

How to Use This Book ................................................... 2
The Latest Science and the Ancient Mystical Traditions ........... 3

Chapter 2  It Is Your Fight—No One Else's ........................... 5

My Strategy for the Best Results ..................................... 5
Get the Best in Modern Medicine ................................... 6
Find the Best Doctor You Can—but Beware of False
Advertising in Medicine ................................................ 7
Do Your Own Research before Deciding on a Doctor .............. 7
Master Roy's Eight-Part Plan for Winning the Big Fight .......... 8
Raising One's Vibes ..................................................... 9
The Amazing Power of Your Body, Mind, and Spirit .............. 10
Laughter Therapy ...................................................... 10
Raise Your Vibes—Be Positive ...................................... 11
Accomplish the First Step First ...................................... 11
Don't Procrastinate .................................................... 12
Find the Best Match Available in Your Situation .................. 13
Sometimes You Try and Try Again ................................... 15

Chapter 3  Diets That Fight the Disease .............................. 20

The Rainbow Diet and the Twelve-Gram Disease-
Starvation Diet .......................................................... 20

Beware of Blindly Followed Protocols..................................23

A Metabolic Disease ..................................................24

A Nobel Prize and Simple Logic ..................................26

Take the Second Step..................................................28

Sugar-Rich Junk Foods, Obesity, and Willpower ....................29

The Macrobiotic Diet ................................................31

Chapter 4   Eat, Drink, and Breathe Clean................................32

Clean Food, Pure Water, and Breathing Deeply ....................33

Picking the Right Supplements....................................33

The Power of Herbs—Don't Overdo It................................34

If You Are Stuck with an Unenlightened Doctor....................35

Building New Good Habits and the Complete Breath ............35

Learn from Your Yoga Teacher or an MD ..........................36

Getting Clean, Healthy Air.........................................36

Getting Clean Air Inside .............................................37

Fasting to Fight the Disease ........................................38

Intermittent Fasting ..................................................38

There Is Hope ...........................................................39

Avoid Environmental Toxins ........................................40

Dr. Ray Sahelian .......................................................41

Eat Clean Food, Drink Pure Water..................................42

Getting Truly Clean Water ...........................................42

Chapter 5   Using Your Mind Positively..................................44

The Difficulty of Changing Belief Systems ....................44

My Brother..................................................45

Enhancing Your Immune System ..................................46

Three Tricks for Better Health......................................47

Beginning the Holistic Battle......................................49

Uniting Body, Mind, and Spirit in One Purpose..................50

Patients with the Best Results ......................................50

Chapter 6   Visualization and Affirmation ............................52

Visualization Made Easy .............................................53

Affirmation and Self-Suggestion................................................ 54
The Power of Affirmations ...................................................... 55
Program Only Positives—Never Negatives .............................. 56
Avoid Negativity—Be Positive ................................................ 57
Begin Combining Your Techniques........................................... 58
Embrace the Simplicity .......................................................... 59

Chapter 7   Causation, Your Spiritual Beliefs, and the "Why Me?"
            Question ................................................................ 61

Higher Power and Spiritual Belief Systems .............................. 61
Why Me?............................................................................... 62
Dealing with Depression........................................................ 63
Causation and the Spiritual Aspect ......................................... 64
The Whole Armor of God....................................................... 65
Causation and Belief Systems................................................. 65

Chapter 8   Prayer and Meditation.............................................. 70

The Huna System of Prayer .................................................... 71
Meditation........................................................................... 73
Life-Force Building Meditations ............................................. 74
Sound and Vibrations in Meditation and Healing..................... 75
Healing Sounds .................................................................... 75
The Science of Cymatics ........................................................ 76
The Power of Words and Intention ......................................... 77
My Shotgun Approach to Self-Healing..................................... 78
Kotodama ............................................................................ 79
Using Sound in Meditation and for Healing............................. 79
Chanting Aum or Amen.......................................................... 80
Load Up with Sound............................................................... 81
Keep Combining Techniques................................................... 82

Chapter 9   Exercising—Western and Eastern ............................. 84

Moving toward Life or Embracing Death ................................. 85
Concerning Life and Death..................................................... 86
Exercising and Support Groups............................................... 86

The Necessity for Support.............................................................. 89

Defeating Depression with Exercise and Positive Activity ...... 89

Develop Your Own Personal Exercise Program....................... 90

Monitor Yourself Honestly........................................................ 91

Western and Eastern Exercise................................................... 91

Use Common Sense and Intuition ........................................... 92

Building Healthy Habits............................................................ 93

Fighting the Disease while Raising Kids and/or Working....... 93

Chapter 10  Radical Remission .................................................... 95

Spontaneous or Radical Remission ......................................... 95

The Nine Principles of Radical Remission.............................. 96

Trust Your Intuition ................................................................. 97

Unblock Any Blockages............................................................ 98

Dealing with the Fear............................................................... 99

The Calling ............................................................................. 100

Your New Belief Systems.........................................................101

Chapter 11  Other Alternative Healing Modalities ...................103

Alternative and Ultra-Alternative/Outlawed Therapies......... 104

The Gerson Therapy ............................................................... 106

Other Alternative Treatments.................................................107

The Baking Soda/Vitamin C Protocol ...................................107

Royal Rife and the High RF Cancer Cure ............................. 108

Be Skeptical.............................................................................110

Desperation .............................................................................111

Use the Power of Belief Wisely ..............................................111

Marijuana.................................................................................112

Chapter 12  Other Alternatives...................................................114

Load Your Shotgun..................................................................115

Use Belief Intelligently ...........................................................116

A Healable Disease ..................................................................116

Chapter 13 Spiritual Healing ................................................118

    Pranic, Psychic, Religious, and Spiritual Healing ..................118

    Genuine Spiritual Healing ....................................................118

    Humans Are Multidimensional Beings ................................119

    The Multidimensional Human Being.................................. 120

    Techniques of Spiritual Healing...........................................121

    A Spiritual Self-Healing Technique...................................... 122

    The Spiritual Reality of Divine Love ................................... 122

    Ruth's Powerful Meditation ................................................ 123

    Ruth Stillman's Meditation ................................................ 123

    Eve's Self-Healing Technique .............................................. 124

    Purification and Cleansing................................................... 126

    Pranic Healing..................................................................... 127

    Psychic Healing .................................................................. 129

    Religious and Spiritual Healing........................................... 129

    Psychic Healing and Spiritual Aid ......................................131

    Receiving Healing ...............................................................131

Chapter 14 Those in Need of Healing—Beware .....................133

    Take Charge!.......................................................................135

Conclusion ...............................................................................137

    Things Keep Getting Better! ............................................... 138

Endnotes ..................................................................................143

# PREFACE

This is a book written by a martial artist, but it is not a book written just for martial artists. It is meant for anyone to use after they get diagnosed with "the big C," to teach them how to fight the battle to win. As a martial artist and expert in self-defense for the disabled, I am always looking for the most effective techniques—those that are most decisive in the shortest possible time. I applied that same logic to this fight.

When I was diagnosed with adenocarcinoma cancer of the bladder on January 9, 2014, I knew I was in the biggest fight of my life because it was the fight *for* my life.

I wrote this book because it is exactly what I wish someone had handed me that first day. It would have greatly improved my life and saved me from weeks of sleepless nights until I finally had a treatment plan, a healing diet, and an exercise program.

If you are a fellow martial artist, you will appreciate my approach: fight to win. My method is to utilize the best in modern medicine combined with the best in diet and exercise, the best of ancient traditional healing practices, the best of modern psychology, and the best from the world of alternative treatments.

If you have been diagnosed, you may have one or several doctors at this point. That is fine. This plan puts *you* in charge of your body, your life, your treatments, and your self-healing. Of course, I cannot guarantee that everyone who reads this book will become free and clear of this disease like I did. Life doesn't work like that; individual results will vary, and this approach requires real self-discipline. However, I do believe with all my heart that in short time it will be proven that those who diligently practice my simple eight-part plan will do significantly statistically better than those patients who passively go through their treatments and don't change their diets or lifestyles.

This is no unfounded guess, but it is a solid assumption based on the work of Dr. Thomas Seyfried, Dr. Dominic D'Agostino, and Dr. Kelly Turner. My eight-part plan is an aggregation of what was already out there. I just put things together into a quick, simple, and well-organized way to fight this disease effectively for those with the will to win.

# CHAPTER 1

# The Diagnosis and the Fight

Absolutely no one who has not heard the words themselves can understand how it feels to hear them. When the doctor says, "You have cancer," your life is irrevocably changed from that moment forward. It will never be the same. But those words do not mean a death sentence. No matter which type of the big C you have, with an early enough diagnosis, you can fight, and in many—if not most—cases, you can win. Even the worst kinds of cancer have a survivability rate. If they tell you that you have one of the worst forms with a survivability rate of 5 percent, you must decide at that moment that you will be in that 5 percent.

New scientific research in this field shows amazing, almost miraculous results. Don't give up hope; decide to fight. Some of these new treatments use modified viruses that were previously dangerous, like polio and HIV. When these altered viruses are introduced in the body, the treatments have incredible results, but they are still experimental.

Your job may be to stay alive until the Food and Drug Administration (FDA) approves some of these new techniques. Unfortunately, that will take more trials and more time. Although there is genuine reason for hope, these treatments are still in the experimental stage and are not currently available. You must deal with the present reality.[1]

Regrettably, the doctor who delivers your diagnosis in most cases will not tell you how to fight, instead only offering what treatments the conventional medical community offers. Most medical doctors have had only one five-hour course in nutrition and are basically ignorant on the

---

[1] **Search Phrase: miraculous cures for cancer + injecting disease.**

1

subject. Most doctors are also not trained in psychology, human motivation, or the power of the subconscious mind. Most physicians are not trained in holistic medicine, functional medicine, or integrative oncology.

How to Use This Book

This is an instructional manual for how to fight this disease and how to activate and supercharge your innate self-healing mechanisms. Every patient should be handed such a book at the time of diagnosis. Instead, after I received a cancer diagnosis, I was in an emotional state of shock for three weeks. It took a simple statement by a nurse for me to snap out of it and begin fighting. When she told me that the mutant cells needed sugar to live and thrive, it woke me up. This was my fight—and fight I could.

This is a simple book about how you can significantly increase the odds that you will win the biggest fight of your life. I give you the tools to fight holistically—with your body, mind, and spirit—but it's your fight. Reading is not enough. I present an eight-part plan, a complete strategy to greatly increase your odds of success.

You must

- go to the suggested sites on the internet and listen to the leading scientists on YouTube;
- take charge of your treatment plan;
- put into practice the techniques presented here; and
- feel like you have taken back control over your body, your life, and the fight for your health.

This book is not academic or scientific in tone or language, but it points you in the right direction to easily do your own research on the internet. I attempt to put things in the simplest, most general terms and allow the reader to dig deeper.

This book is designed to be read with your computer, laptop, smartphone, or whatever electronic device you use so you can use Google (or any decent search engine) to research the subject being discussed.

At the bottom of the page, I give you the specific internet address or search phrase(s) to type into your search engine.

I may not be a doctor or a scientist, but I can direct you to YouTube videos where you can hear for yourself what the leaders in these fields are currently teaching. Fighting this disease holistically, metabolically, and in an integrated way is a dynamic new field of study that is rapidly moving forward. The best way to keep up is on the internet.

## The Latest Science and the Ancient Mystical Traditions

Although I try to get good scientific or medical sources for all the strategies and techniques presented here, not everything I teach comes from today's science or modern medicine. I was taught mouth-to-ear by a variety of teachers in the ancient mystical tradition.

If you enter "mystical traditions" in your internet search engine, you will find that many philosophies and almost all religions have a mystical, esoteric side that is not taught in the outer teachings for the masses. This knowledge has always been taught directly to the initiates from the mouth of the teacher to the ear of the student in a direct transmission of information.[2] During my life, I have been extremely fortunate to study under several spiritual teachers; they include the following:

- martial artists Master Jack Johns and Master Robert Quinn
- nationally renowned psychic, metaphysician, and author Evelyn Monahan
- Esoteric Section–trained Theosophist Ruth Stillman
- mystical Priest of the Liberal Catholic Church Father Brian Brinkerhoff
- Buddhist healer Dr. Gail Pierce
- Métis shaman (medicine woman) and best-selling author Grandmother Evelyn Eaton
- Northern Paiute shaman (medicine man) Grandfather Raymond Stone

Influential twentieth-century author Aldous Huxley wrote about this mystical tradition at the heart of most philosophies and religions in *The*

---

[2] **Search Phrase: mystical tradition.**

*Perennial Philosophy.* Some of my teachers referred to it as *the ancient wisdom.*

There are continual mystical traditions that have been passed down verbally for hundreds or thousands of years, depending upon which culture you study. I was the recipient of such knowledge from several of my teachers.

Throughout my lifetime I've studied the power of the human mind. I majored in symbolic anthropology and minored in psychology in college, but also studied outside academia—including taking an offshoot course of Silva Mind Control called Phase Five and a twenty-hour course in clinical hypnosis.

For three years, I studied with Grandmother Eve and Grandfather Raymond, and I wrote my honors thesis about the effect of Christianity on traditional Northern Paiute ritual practice: *The Shaman between Worlds* by R. E. Day, Jr. (available on Amazon.com). However, I am not writing this book for academics or in an academic style. I am writing this as a free and clear cancer survivor who is passing on a program that worked for me, a program that combines wisdom and techniques from

- the mystical tradition,
- modern psychology,
- modern medicine,
- dietary knowledge, and
- exercise physiology.

Because I draw from the mystical traditions, not everything presented here can be easily verified by a scientific source on the internet. Some is based on my experience studying shamanism and other mystical traditions.

What I learned with the Northern Paiutes about spiritual and psychological healing has been practiced continuously for at least thirty thousand years.

I studied other spiritual traditions as well, especially the Western esoteric Christian practices and the Eastern mystical spiritual traditions of China, Japan, and India. What is presented here is the latest scientific research you can find on the internet combined with techniques from several mystical traditions that are thousands of years old.

# CHAPTER 2

# It Is Your Fight—No One Else's

You alone can decide how you will fight for your life and with how much passion and ferocity. You can be a passive onlooker in your medical treatment, or you can take the reins and fight holistically by activating your self-healing mechanisms and supercharging your immune system.

There will be some readers who are already familiar with the tools I describe and know how to use them. Unfortunately, most of the people who are diagnosed will have no idea how to fight or will be in such a state of shock they might not immediately remember what they do know, which is what happened to me. Let's look at how you can fight starting that first day.

My Strategy for the Best Results

- Get the best medical advice you can and decide on your course of treatment.
- Use your mind positively and creatively.
- Stop consuming sugar and most carbohydrates, which all become sugar in your body. Feed your body the right nutrition while you starve the disease.
- Build up the oxygen level in your blood and build your life force with deep breathing.
- Exercise and keep fit.
- Use the body-mind-spirit connection to heal yourself.

## Get the Best in Modern Medicine

You must immediately look at what your doctor offers you in the form of orthodox medicine. What is his or her treatment plan, and do you agree with it?

My way of fighting is a simple combination. I believe in seeking the absolute best modern medical help available and supplementing that with the most current knowledge of nutrition and exercise physiology, the most effective techniques from modern psychology, and the best of ancient traditional medicine and practices. From the very beginning of this journey, you must not be passive; you must take control.

You—and only you—must oversee all your treatments. You must investigate the success rates for your specific situation, decide which procedures and treatments being offered make the most sense, and choose which *you* will undergo. Any doctor who disagrees with this approach and thinks he or she doesn't need to consult with you or seek your approval before poisoning you with chemotherapy or radiation needs to be replaced immediately with someone who understands this is your life and your decision about a treatment plan.

I will provide you with a plan for self-healing to supplement what the doctors do. You must research your specific type and stage of cancer and the success rates for chemotherapy, radiation, and surgery for that specific manifestation. You may need immediate treatment, but it still needs to be explained fully to you in a way you understand. And it is still and always your decision. It is your body.

Oncologists are plentiful, and in most locations, they can be easily replaced by one who will truly listen to you. If you have a doctor who ignores your input, you must find a better physician. Just call your previous doctor's office and tell them you're getting a second opinion and please forward your files to the new physician's office. It is that easy to change doctors.

Find the Best Doctor You Can—but Beware
of False Advertising in Medicine

If you can, find a medical doctor who is well respected and is truly

- an integrative oncologist (who utilizes modern medicine along with diet, exercise, and a holistic approach),[3] or
- an oncologist or other specialist who is philosophically holistic, or
- a doctor truly practicing functional medicine (who is not a greedy quack—there appears to be an overabundance of such).

Such doctors will probably be very receptive to the strategies and techniques taught in this book.

Beware of hospitals and doctors who use some of the above terms rather loosely. When holistic medicine first became the next craze in medicine, I saw hospital after hospital proclaim in large signs, they were practicing holistic medicine when they were not. Offering a couple of outpatient yoga classes was better than not offering outpatient yoga classes, but that does not mean the doctors were practicing holistic medicine because they absolutely were not. I know because I personally investigated at different hospitals. Medicine is just as susceptible to fads and the use of misleading advertising as any other aspect of society.

Do Your Own Research before Deciding on a Doctor

It might be best if you could find a doctor who is practicing integrative oncology or is at least holistic. Possibly you could use a doctor who is ethically practicing functional medicine.

Good luck because finding an integrative oncologist or holistic oncologist may be much harder to find than you might expect. Integrative oncologists are rare, and they may be so far away it may not be logistically practical to utilize them. I didn't even know the field of integrative oncology existed when I was diagnosed.

You—and if possible, your loved ones—must do a lot of research

---

[3] **Search Phrase: integrative oncology.**

before deciding on someone practicing holistic, functional, or concierge medicine. Although I love the idea of the doctor and other specialists spending hours with the patient on the first visit—and I love the idea of an MD working with a team of alternative and holistic practitioners—my research indicated that usually means spending a lot of your own cash up front.

I saw one review of such a practice where a patient had spent $5,000 and felt like they had gotten zero results. This is an all-too-common experience.

Although I would like to believe that the majority of medical doctors are ethical and well-meaning healers, watching the news tells you that there is a percentage that is not. How many doctors are genuine healers and how many are unethical money-grubbers is something readers will have to decide for themselves.

Just be warned, do a ton of research—both word of mouth and computer research—and read multiple reviews on the internet before you spend thousands of dollars. I am extremely wary of doctors who jump on the latest fad or craze in medicine.

Always consider and research the doctors' backgrounds. What schools did they go to? What kinds of medicine have they practiced or specialized in? Are they certified by the relevant medical boards? Have they been sued much for malpractice? Have many complaints been filed against them? Time is always precious, and you don't want to waste it on quacks or money-grubbers.

## Master Roy's Eight-Part Plan for Winning the Big Fight

- Combine what *you decide to utilize* from the best of conventional modern medical testing and treatment with
- diets that starve or fight the disease;
- exercises—both traditional and modern; combining yoga, Tai Chi, or Qi Gong deep breathing exercises (all believed to build up your life force), which physiologically raise the oxygen level in your blood along with modern cardiovascular exercise and weight training;
- visualization;

- positive affirmation;
- meditation;
- prayer for others and yourself; and
- raising your vibes—using sound, laughter, love, and nature.

If you are agnostic or atheist and don't believe in the efficacy of prayer, just ignore the prayer part for now.

## Raising One's Vibes

Most of these eight parts seem self-explanatory, so let's begin by clarifying the last one.

- On a molecular, atomic, and subatomic level, everything in the universe is in motion, everything vibrates, and absolutely all natural objects have a frequency or combination of frequencies.[4]
- As they taught in the sixties and seventies, you can raise your personal vibes—your individual frequency—with your intentions, actions, emotions, and practices.
- On an emotional and psychological level, your vibes are how you feel and what energy you exude.
- When you are happy and positive, you feel and exude differently than when you are depressed and negative.
- Your emotions and psychological states have a definite impact on your body and, most importantly, on your immune system.
- The posture, body language, and movement of someone who is healthy, positive, vibrant, and energetic is vastly different from someone who is sad, depressed, negative, and unenergetic.
- By exercising, breathing deeply, eating healthily, and having a positive attitude, one activates the body-mind-spirit connection to raise one's vibes, which physically boosts the immune system. This is much superior to being depressed, getting no exercise, and eating a lot of unhealthy food and sugar, which inhibits the immune system and feeds the disease.

---

[4] **Search Phrases: everything vibrates, everything has frequency, all natural objects have a frequency.**

## The Amazing Power of Your Body, Mind, and Spirit

In general, much of modern medicine concentrates on the symptoms of the body, commonly ignoring the last two of the body-mind-spirit trinity that makes up the human being. This book teaches you to utilize the truly amazing power of each. You may not have access to an integrative or holistic oncologist—I certainly didn't—and you may have to do some or most of this *on your own.*

Although it would be best to have an integrative/holistic oncologist, it may not be logistically possible for you. It is best to be part of a positive team approach, but when it comes down to reality, your doctor doesn't have to agree with all of this—or even know about it. All he or she must do is his or her job, utilizing those practices that *you* agree to.

Your physicians may be excellent at what they do, but they may know less about nutrition than you do. They may understand little about the vast power of the motivated conscious, subconscious, and superconscious of the strong-willed self-healer.[5]

## Laughter Therapy

Norman Cousins, a famous magazine publisher in his day, wrote *Anatomy of an Illness*, in which he describes using laughter therapy and how he laughed himself back to health by watching movies by the Marx Brothers.[6]

Anything you learn here or already know about how to stay positive and happy, do it and raise your vibes. You must move from depressed to positive, from passive to active, from feeling helpless to feeling in control. You must work to raise your vibes. The posture, movement, physiology, and immune functions of a positive and happy individual are different from those of a depressed and negative person.

You can find talks by Norman Cousins about laughter therapy on YouTube, and his book is still for sale.

---

[5] Search Phrases: **integrative oncology, superconscious.**
[6] Search Phrases: **Norman Cousins, laughter therapy, and *Anatomy of an Illness.***

## Raise Your Vibes—Be Positive

In this fight, you must take advantage of every opportunity available to you to raise your vibes to a higher and more positive state of mind by

- communing with nature,
- singing or chanting in the bathtub,
- watching your favorite comedies or comedians,
- hugs and affection from loved ones and for adults, sexual intimacy,
- meditating,
- praying,
- doing whatever makes you feel better,
- doing whatever makes you feel happy and positive, and
- raising your vibes to the highest level you can—every day.

Fight this fight with a positive attitude. Absorb the beauty of Mother Nature. Mystics believe bathing every day cleans more than just your physical body and is highly advised. Use that time in the tub or shower to sing or even better to chant. Sound can be incredibly healing. Find as much joy as you can in life. With every medical victory and every improvement, let your confidence grow—and find more and more joy.

## Accomplish the First Step First

For your own peace of mind, you must immediately accomplish step 1 of my eight-part plan. Some people eschew modern medicine and will choose to take a completely alternative route. Those who take this approach must do a lot of research, keep great discipline with diet and exercise, have true faith in what they are doing, and maintain a truly disciplined spiritual practice. I would certainly never advise anyone to take this path, but I acknowledge with great respect the small percentage of people who do this successfully. However, it would be foolhardy and extremely dangerous for the average American. Most modern Americans need medical testing and answers, scientific knowledge, and a treatment plan that utilizes what they intelligently choose from the best of modern medicine.

Consider the doctors and hospitals you have access to, investigate which have the best modern medical care and the best results for your specific illness. Find those who you philosophically agree with on the plan and type of care. Find the best medical testing and treatment available, and if you agree with their plan, start immediately.

Don't be passive! Investigate, do your own research, be in charge, and make intelligent choices based on your own research.

You—or a loved one—must do research on the internet and ask anyone you can for the names of the leading doctors and professors treating your issues. If you aren't satisfied with your first choice, don't be afraid to go somewhere else. I did. Get second and third opinions when appropriate.

## Don't Procrastinate

The sooner you start treatment, the better. If I remember correctly, a CNN *Healthwatch* segment reported that Taiwan had a 25 percent better cure rate than the United States using the same treatments (using only modern medicine and not traditional treatments). The only difference was the start of medical treatment.

In the United States, after you get diagnosed, they set up appointments. You go home for two or three weeks of absolutely miserable sleepless nights. In Taiwan, the day you are diagnosed, you walk down the hall to another office and begin testing and treatment.

In Taiwan, there is no two or three weeks waiting to begin treatment, which results in a 25 percent better cure rate. In the United States, your mind is spinning like the exercise wheel in a hamster's cage after you hear the diagnosis, all the dire warnings, and all the bad news over and over and over again in an endless loop before your first appointment.

For me, that hamster wheel spun every sleepless night, and it didn't stop turning until I was fighting on many fronts. When I knew I was fighting the good fight, I could go to sleep tired each night.

## Find the Best Match Available in Your Situation

Get the absolute best modern medical testing and treatment available to you that match your situation, your personality, your logistical situation, and your way of fighting. Since the standard, conventional treatments for most forms of this disease are either surgical or involve chemotherapy and/or radiation, which are extremely toxic and may have a high or low percentage of success, *you* must decide on what therapies *you* choose.

The beginning of many treatments will be further diagnostics to see exactly what you are dealing with. The fact that you are being seen and tested—the reality of taking physical actions—should make you feel better psychologically. Sometimes surgery is needed immediately to save your life. Sometimes there is more time to plan.

Before you accept chemotherapy or radiation or go under the scalpel, do your own research. The doctors will tell you that some forms of this disease are highly susceptible to being healed by chemo or radiation, and others are not. When you are told this, get specific statistics. If the cure rate is very high in your specific situation, make your decision, do your research, and decide what's best for you.

In my case, what they found needed to be surgically removed immediately. When I heard what was there, and only there, it made sense to me to get it out and get it all out quickly. Chemo or radiation was a discussion for a later day, an afterthought. However, at the beginning it felt like everything moved so slowly.

When you are ill, you want to get well immediately. This is not the twenty-four-hour flu; this is the fight of your life.

There are myriad manifestations of this disease, but speaking generally, for many decades, conventional medical practice had three and only three weapons: the scalpel, radiation, and chemotherapy. You must talk to your physicians and loved ones, do research on your specific condition, and decide what is right for you. Truly miraculous-seeming research is being done, and there is reason for great hope and optimism in the future. However, you must deal with the reality of the moment. If all a doctor knows how to do is use chemo or radiation, they may try to use it when it is not very applicable to your specific case. Do research and ask your doctors for the success rate of any treatments or procedures.

Always ask your doctor to define and explain in understandable language all medical terms, tests, and procedures. Be sure you clearly understand your treatment options. Your definition of success will be healed, free and clear, healthy, and back to normal. Many oncologists' definition of success in any given situation might be much more limited than yours. It is up to you to ask and find out these things.

Some forms of the disease are highly receptive to one or more of these three treatments. Others are not as receptive to one or more of these therapies, but if that's all the doctor was taught to do, they will probably try to do what they know.[7] In some instances, after you do your research, you may decide not to be poisoned by radiation or chemo and try alternative therapies that may be effective. I believe in getting the absolute best medical care applicable in combination with the best alternatives.

Before agreeing to any treatment plan, you must research the doctor and the proposed treatment plan by word of mouth, the internet, and asking your other doctors and anyone else you know in the medical field. Get multiple opinions, do your research, and check their reviews online.[8] Just because a doctor or a friend says something, it doesn't mean it is absolutely correct or suits your specific situation. In my experience, reputations in medicine at the local hospital level should not be blindly trusted.

You must do the research, but you might not get it right the first time. You may not get the right doctor or treatment plan on the first try—or even the second. You must try to stay positive and be patient at the same time. If the first place you go isn't a good fit, go somewhere else. Do more research. Keep trying until you find the right fit. Good, competent doctors respect patients who want second opinions.

Although medicine is practiced at a very high level in many American institutions, the overall medical system is broken in many ways and is in need of repair. Don't get too frustrated by the broken system or the wrong doctor. Try to keep a positive attitude—even when dealing with insurance or medical bureaucracy. It will not be easy, and at times, it may be extremely difficult, but try to stay positive.

---

[7] **Search Phrases: your diagnosis (your specific type and stage of cancer) + chemotherapy, your diagnosis + radiation, your diagnosis + surgery, your diagnosis + holistic therapies.**

[8] **Search Phrases: your doctor's name + reviews, your doctor's practice + reviews.**

I did a lot of research, and so did my insurance company's nurse, and it still all went wrong for me the first time.


## Sometimes You Try and Try Again

I don't want this book to be about me; I want it to be about how *you* fight. There is, however, the reader's natural curiosity plus the need of using my personal experiences as an example, which necessitates divulging some biographical material. After my diagnosis, I did not immediately get the best conventional help. I took a few missteps, which cost me precious time and all the attendant anxiety.

Decades ago, I was in an industrial demolition mishap. A building fell, and four of us rode a broken crane boom down about seven stories. Two of my fellow workers died and one was DOA at the hospital but was revived. I had a broken back, a spinal cord injury where the 12th thoracic and 1st lumbar vertebrae merged into one busted-up vertebrae. My paralysis was lower on the front and right, higher in the back and left, going on a diagonal across my body from almost waist level in the back on my left to the top of my right thigh. The nerves to my bladder were severely damaged, resulting in a neurogenic bladder. Facing the various options open to me, I went with the suprapubic catheter: a tube going from outside of the body directly into the bladder. As an athletic and sexual person, it seemed much better than the alternative of a condom catheter.

For decades, everything went well. I learned the procedure of taking the suprapubic catheter out and replacing it with a new one every two or three months. Although it was considered minor surgery, it was important to me to be independent. For part of that time, I was living in a remote log cabin, which was very rustic and had extremely limited facilities, and any medical help was a long drive away if there was an emergency. Because I took care of almost everything, I seldom saw a urologist.

However, from the time I was eighteen, every urologist I saw warned me about the eventual danger of bladder cancer due to the irritation of an indwelling catheter. One of them delivered a dire warning: if I got it to act quickly, it could be fatal in a short time. Although that warning had been issued decades before my diagnosis by a different urologist, it was one of the rotating thoughts that inhabited the hamster wheel every sleepless night before I took charge.

For decades, there were no serious problems with the suprapubic catheter other than the occasional bladder infection, which is par for the course for most paraplegics. Then, in the winter of 2014, there were problems. The catheter wasn't draining properly. Before Christmas, I knew I needed help. My urologist insisted on waiting until after Christmas for an exploratory procedure. He scheduled me to come in for the procedure on January 8. On January 9, I was officially diagnosed over the phone with bladder cancer, but I knew it on January 8.

On January 8, some abnormal-looking tissue came out during the procedure and fell on the white cloth covering the surgical table. Everyone froze for a moment. The doctor and I looked at each other. After a second or two, he said that he would be remiss in his duties if he didn't have it tested. I agreed that he would be. I came out of the procedure in a state of shock. I was white as a ghost. My brother looked at me and knew something was wrong. When he asked, all I would say was that it wasn't good.

On January 8, it would have been hard for me to believe the circuitous route I would take. I eventually went to the right institution, with the right doctor, and went on an extreme diet for six months, had two surgeries, and was free and clear within one year—without radiation or chemotherapy. Five years later, I continue to be free and clear.

My insurance company's case manager who was an RN did extensive research for me, and I did research too. It seemed to indicate that MD Anderson in Houston had the absolute best results in treating bladder cancer. My urologist in Atlanta agreed it was an excellent facility. The tests done in Atlanta indicated I had a golf ball-sized tumor in my bladder. The type was adenocarcinoma, which doesn't always stay put. As far as diagnoses go, there are better—and there are many worse. Every indication in the x-rays was that the mutant cells were only in my bladder. I felt like I could hear the clock ticking. Things needed to happen quickly. Reservations were made for me to go to MD Anderson, and absolutely everything went wrong. It was one of the worst medical experiences of my life.

My insurance company did a great job throughout the process—with a few exceptions. To start, the insurance company wouldn't pay for my brother to go with me. I'm a very independent person in a wheelchair but traveling from Atlanta to Houston and with all the meetings and tests, I wanted someone to be with me. That was my first complaint. The second was that the company they used to arrange ground transportation and hotels was one of the most inefficient companies I'd ever seen. Logistically, everything went wrong.

When we got to the Houston airport, the ground transportation never arrived. Finally, we made our own arrangements. We were taken to the Marriott at MD Anderson where we'd been told our reservations were, but they were actually at a different Marriott, which was a few miles away. So, it went, hour after hour, waiting and waiting, mistake after mistake. When these things happen, you must try to remain as positive as possible and not let them get you down.

The guy who scheduled us at MD Anderson was new, and there were a lot of communication problems. I arrived on a Thursday and saw a doctor on Friday. The doctor I was assigned was going on a holiday for a wedding in India and would be gone for three weeks. That made no sense to me. Why let me come from Atlanta to see a doctor who was going on vacation? That seemed stupid to me.

I handed the disappearing doctor a disk with my medical information. In my previous experiences at the Mayo Clinic in Jacksonville, when I handed world-famous surgeon Dr. Mary O'Connor a disk of information, she would put in into their computer system as she continued talking to me. This doctor took the disk I handed him and set it aside. The idea that I had been assigned a doctor leaving on holiday for three weeks seemed insensitive to my needs and bad medicine. Then, there were the medical tests—or lack thereof.

The only tests the world-famous MD Anderson could accomplish that day were simple blood and urine tests. They were going to do an MRI, but that was a half-day wasted fiasco. Years earlier, I had a benign polyp/tumor removed from my sinuses at Emory Hospital in Atlanta, and they left a screw inside my head during the surgery. I told everybody at Anderson about it, every step of the way. The fourth time, and many hours into this process, I repeated my warning about the screw as they were wheeling me into the MRI.

The techs stopped the gurney and asked me what year. I told them, and they made a phone call. The IV drip was finished. I was about five feet from the door—on the gurney for another half hour—when the word came down to abort. We went back to the hotel, amazed that MD Anderson could have such a great reputation and be such an absolute disaster for me.

My insurance company's nurse back in Atlanta told us to stay put; she was sure they could do better, and she could get things on track. On Monday, things were the same. It would be a minimum of three weeks before treatment or surgery.

When we tried to fly out, a massive snowstorm had hit Atlanta. Delta had quit flying, but we caught United through Chicago to Atlanta. We tried to get home from the airport that night, but the city was totally shut down. We spent the night in the airport. Delta was great. I no longer had a ticket out of Atlanta, but they let me spend the night in the less crowded secure area. After thirty hours at the airport, we finally made it home.

We had done our research, and we thought we had chosen the right place. It was supposed to be the best place in the country—if not the world—and it had been an absolute disaster for me. In Houston while on the phone with the nurse in Atlanta, I got the information that would change everything for me. I was considered allergic to iodine and couldn't do some tests. If I couldn't do the MRI because of the screw, what other tests could they do?

The nurse told me they could do a PET scan. I was unfamiliar with that test so she explained that a PET scan required hooking up the patient to an IV bag of glucose and seeing where it goes because cancer lives off sugar. (It's a little more complicated than that, but her basic idea was correct. An FDG PET scan does reveal excess glucose consumption, which reveals the location of the cancer.)

I asked her to repeat what she had said, and she repeated everything, including the part I was waiting on: cancer lives off sugar. I quit eating the chocolate sundaes I'd been eating every night, and I quit eating all sweets immediately.

I had difficulty believing that not a single person in the medical community had mentioned the fact that the disease lives off sugar. They told me I had a golf ball-sized adenocarcinoma tumor, but not a single medical professional told me it lived off sugar so maybe now would be a good time to cut out sugar. Not a single word. It was *my* questions about the PET scan that finally elicited that knowledge.

Don't feed the disease—go low carb! Eliminate all sugar and almost all starches from your diet immediately!

The first thing I did when I got home was to go to my computer and put in "diets that defeat or fight cancer." My world was about to change for the second time in a month, but this time, it was changing for the better.

I found YouTube videos by Dr. Thomas Seyfried and Dominic D'Agostino that literally changed my life.[9]

---

[9] **Search Phrases: sugar + cancer, FDG PET Scan + glucose, diets that fight cancer, Diets that defeat cancer, Diets that starve cancer; On YouTube: #TalkingKeto: Professor Tom Seyfried, and Starving Cancer: Dominic D'Agostino at TEDx.**

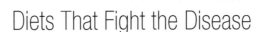

# CHAPTER 3

## Diets That Fight the Disease

### The Rainbow Diet and the Twelve-Gram Disease-Starvation Diet

I found several diets of interest. There is the rainbow diet out of England. My understanding is it was developed by a father who was determined that his daughter not die from the tumors in her brain. He researched and investigated foods that fight this disease or boost the immune system. I was impressed.

The rainbow diet emphasizes the effects of the nutrients that cause the colors in foods, in healing the human body, specifically in fighting this disease. His daughter got well, and if you are not going to take the more direct—but more disciplined—disease-starvation approach, I highly recommend his book and approach to fighting this disease. Go to your search engine and type in "rainbow diet to fight cancer." The approach I decided upon was different. Instead of eating to fight the disease, I choose eating to starve the disease, based on the 1931 Nobel Prize–winning work of Dr. Otto Warburg.[10]

In 1931, Warburg proved that the metabolism of mutant cells and normal cells are different in many ways. One aspect of his Nobel Prize–winning work indicated that mutant cells live on and are dependent upon sugar (glucose and glycine) for their survival. Now called *the Warburg effect,* when deprived of glucose (and glycine)—the body's normal fuel

---

[10] **Search Phrases: Nobel Prize + Otto Warburg, the Rainbow Diet to Fight Cancer, the 12 grams of carbs a day diet to starve cancer.**

source—the mutant cells starve because they cannot live on the body's alternative fuel of ketones (as made famous in the Atkins diet).

This is referred to by some as using the Warburg effect to fight cancer on a metabolic level. I call it the (Warburg effect) twelve-gram disease-starvation diet because that is what it is. By using the Warburg effect and limiting one's intake to twelve grams of carbohydrates a day, the mutant cells starve. The anecdotal evidence says either of two things will happen at that point. The mutant cells of the disease either disappear, or dangerous tumors are transformed into benign tumors, which is what happened with me.

Although much research is being done using the ketogenic diet to combat a variety of illnesses, do not expect most doctors to know about this.

Doctors at Johns Hopkins have been using the ketogenic diet to successfully fight childhood epilepsy for decades. Some people eventually observed that, besides curing childhood epileptic seizures, a strict ketogenic diet deprives mutant cells of their food—glucose. Anecdotal evidence repeatedly shows that when mutant cells are deprived of sugars and must live off the alternative fuel, ketones, the mutant cells starve, and tumors either disappear or become benign.

In anecdotal literature on the twelve-gram disease-starvation diet also known as—*the ketogenic diet to starve cancer*—when followed strictly, either of two things will happen. The mutant cells are replaced by healthy cells—tumors go from bad to benign—or the mutant cells just disappear. The diet requires an extreme amount of self-discipline.

You must do your own research on the internet before going further. Get online. If you are not a computer person, get one of your grandkids or pay a neighborhood kid to get you online and go to YouTube. I cannot possibly explain this subject as well as two of the leading scientists in this field.

Go to YouTube and find the short talk called "Starving Cancer: Dominic D'Agostino at TEDx at Tampa Bay." This ten-and-a-half-minute talk is a good introduction to the field. Next, find the video "#TalkingKeto:

Professor Tom Seyfried." It is fifteen minutes that can change your life. I would watch both these videos a couple of times before moving forward.[11]

If you watch these videos and absorb the basics, you will know more about the subject than most practicing physicians in the United States. This is what you will be up against as you take charge of your conventional treatment plan.

One oncologist I really like told me that if you could starve cancer cells surely, they would have taught him that in med school. Wrong! Interested scientists could have deduced that mutant cells cannot survive on ketones since the Nobel Prize in the 1930s, but the idea of a metabolic cause, treatment, and cure for cancer did not fit the prevalent theories of the time and was not adopted. Professors didn't teach it, so doctors didn't learn it. This has continued for decades. Today, there remains absolutely no *financial* incentive for medical schools, hospitals, pharmaceutical companies, or oncology physicians to promote a metabolic, dietary treatment for this disease, and it has not become prevalent as it should have.

Listen carefully to what Dr. Seyfried says concerning this. If the med schools don't teach it, most doctors don't know it. Also listen to his sadness talking about patients who die unnecessarily from the toxicity of chemo and radiation.

Do your own research. Look up "12 grams of carbs a day to starve cancer" on YouTube, and these sites will explain how they are using the Warburg effect to starve cancer cells. If you go to the scholarly articles on the Warburg effect, they will be very technical. Look at the bottom of some of the best articles; they may lead you to the less scientific and easier-to-understand articles or talks on YouTube.

In a ketogenic diet, your ketones—your glucose replacement—come from fats and oils. This is a very significant change for the human body. It is changing the fuel it runs on. Read and research. The change from sugar to ketones can be very rough on your body for several days—so learn what to expect ahead of time.

Don't feed your disease. Quit eating sugar, including all starches, and most fruits! Do not use artificial sweeteners; they are carcinogenic. Instead, use stevia, which comes from a green leafy plant!

---

[11] **Search Phrases: Starving Cancer: Dominic D'Agostino at TEDx at Tampa Bay, #TalkingKeto: Professor Tom Seyfried."**

This book was written to be simple and easy to read; you must do your own in-depth study. Get on the internet. This stuff is not hard to find. If you haven't already done so, start with "diets that fight cancer," "ketogenic diet to starve cancer" and "twelve grams of carbs to starve cancer." [12]

The ketogenic diet has been studied since the 1920s, and its current form was developed at Johns Hopkins to fight childhood epileptic seizures. It was successful. Dr. Thomas Seyfried explains how they still cannot explain exactly how the ketogenic diet suppresses or cures a person's seizures, but they can explain exactly how the ketogenic diet starves cancer cells.

A study was commissioned by the US Navy because a certain percentage of Navy SEALs was having seizures during long underwater missions using rebreathers. Dominic D'Agostino did this research, and the ketogenic diet was successful for the SEALs.

Both doctors heard of the other result—that the ketogenic diet starved cancer cells—and did their own research. You must watch and really listen to the short talks by Seyfried and D'Agostino on YouTube. Listening to Seyfried and D'Agostino will give you the knowledge and strength you'll need to stand up against a doctor who may want to give you a toxic therapy you disagree with. There are many sites dedicated to and books written about this subject. [13]

## Beware of Blindly Followed Protocols

As a previous oncology patient, I must warn you to beware of doctors who blindly follow protocols. I had a highly respected oncologist in Atlanta try to circumvent the treatment plan of the Mayo Clinic. While I was using the twelve-gram disease-starvation diet, I had two surgeries. After that,

---

[12] **Search Phrase: the ketogenic diet to starve cancer.**
[13] **Internet sites on the subject:**
*KetoDietResource.com* and *KetoNutrition.org*
**Books on the subject:**
*Cancer as a Metabolic Disease* by Thomas Seyfried
*The Cantin Ketogenic Diet* by Elaine Cantin (dairy-free)
*Fight Cancer with a Ketogenic Diet* by Ellen Davis

I was declared free and clear. My doctors at Mayo took the no-radiation, no-chemo, wait-and-watch approach. I would be tested regularly.

After my second surgery, my oncologist in Atlanta scheduled a chest tube and four months of chemo all on her own. I went down to Mayo, and they tested. On their advice, I canceled the chest tube and the four months of toxic poisoning. After the second surgery, I was weak and needed to recover—not be poisoned.

Dr. Seyfried will repeatedly say he can't tell you exactly how the ketogenic diet stops seizures, but he can explain exactly how it starves and defeats cancer. The formula is simple: switch to a healthy ketogenic diet, limit your intake of all carbs to twelve grams a day or less, and live on this extreme Atkins-style diet to starve/transform bad cells into good cells.

Do your research. This is no small transition and no small change in diet. The change in your body's fuel can be very rough for three days or so. Do your research, and you will not be surprised. Your body is changing its fuel source. At times during the transition, I felt like my heart was racing. Experiences will vary by individual. You must be extremely disciplined and work very hard to get the proper nutrition while keeping all cumulative carbs to twelve grams each day. This is not easy, and those without the needed self-discipline should look at the rainbow diet or similar alternatives.[14]

## A Metabolic Disease

I ordered a book from England by Ellen Davis entitled *Fight Cancer with a Ketogenic Diet*. I took a thumb drive and had it printed in book form at Kinko's. I read the book, but in all honesty, I mostly just used the charts. I kept it simple. To starve the bad cells, you must eat no more than twelve grams of carbohydrates a day. If you can do that, and live on a healthy ketogenic diet, the anecdotal evidence says the bad cells will starve to death.

Interested scientists should have known the mechanics of this since 1931. I don't think anybody is saying there is some intentional conspiracy to suppress a metabolic, dietary cure. I think it was just easier for the med schools to ignore and dismiss this approach because it did not fit

---

[14] **Search Phrase: Keto support groups.**

the prevalent theory for the cause or the standard treatments for cancer at that time. It was easy for them to ignore for decades because it wasn't surgery, chemo, or radiation. Their disease model at the time was not metabolic, and to many, it still is not. Now there is much evidence to the contrary and things are rapidly and dynamically changing.[15]

Because the metabolic approach did not fit the standard theory or practice of the time, it was ignored:

- Medical schools have not taught this to doctors.
- It has almost been a secret in the very medical community that should have embraced it in 1932.
- This is an absolute disgrace. The entire medical community should become aware of this and ashamed of it—and work to correct this.

I am not saying there was ever any organized, intentional effort to suppress the idea of a metabolic cause and treatment for this disease; this approach to the disease was easy to ignore or dismiss in 1931 because it wasn't mainstream and didn't fit their theories and practices. For decades, it remained buried and ignored. However, today the cat is out of the bag. The information is out there. Unfortunately, medicine in the United States is profit-driven, and there is no profit for the pharmaceutical companies if people adopt this diet and get well. Hospitals would make much less money from cancer patients; pharmaceutical companies would make nothing off this diet. Billions of dollars would be lost by pharmaceutical companies, hospitals, and doctors if this diet became a standard conventional treatment for oncologists.

There is still no definitive double-blind human study of patients testing the twelve-grams disease-starvation diet versus the conventional chemo and radiation treatments. Dr. Seyfried argues that each case is so individual that the standard double-blind studies would be difficult.

Maybe there could be a voluntary registry on the internet where those who implemented this diet could register their diagnoses and results. As the numbers grow to be significant, scientists could compare our

---

[15] **Search Phrase: Is cancer a metabolic disease?**

results against the standard cure rates and see how much better we do by starving the mutant cells than they currently do by poisoning them.

There are more and more scientific studies that indicate the ketogenic diet is effective in combination with modern treatments for a variety of problems, and some people think public demand is so high that double-blind tests with the twelve-gram diet are eventually coming.

One problem is that most of the institutions that usually run such studies have an obvious financial disincentive. If this was a universally accepted, highly effective treatment, it would mean the real loss of millions of dollars to pharmaceutical companies and hospitals. Do not fool yourself into thinking this is insignificant; we are talking millions and possibly billions of dollars.

Although none of these three pillars of modern medicine—med schools and the doctors they produce, hospitals, and pharmaceutical companies—did anything for decades about arranging a good double-blind study comparing patients using only modern medicine compared to patients using modern medicine while on a strict ketogenic diet, the anecdotal success is demanding such studies and medical recognition.

## A Nobel Prize and Simple Logic

It is hard to argue with a Nobel Prize and simple, clean logic, but the medical community has done it for decades while hundreds of thousands of patients died without trying this therapy, decade after decade, year after deadly year.

I love the good doctors—those who are actual healers. However, many of the best doctors, at the best institutions, with the best healing intentions, know nothing about the ketogenic diet. That's why you must do your own research and map out the treatment regime you desire.

Don't let the intrinsic greed and self-interest inherent in some parts of the American medical community cost you your life. Some of the best institutions, like the Mayo Clinic or Johns Hopkins, or places like the Cancer Treatment Centers, which are holistic as well as conventional, allow the patient to be in charge of their treatment. You may go to an excellent hospital, and your surgeons may know nothing about the ketogenic diet to fight cancer, but their nutritionists certainly will. Wherever you go for treatment, ask for their dietician/nutritionist to immediately become involved in your care. If their dietician/nutritionist is not familiar with the ketogenic twelve-gram disease-starvation diet or the rainbow diet, you may need to go to a better institution.

In my opinion, the Mayo Clinic and Johns Hopkins systems represent the best hospitals and the most complete medical facilities in the United States. I can't pretend to know all the hospitals; this is just from my personal knowledge and experience. There are several of these spread around the country, and they have outreach programs where they partner with regional/local facilities.

There are also centers that specialize in this disease and are very holistic in nature. Although I went to Mayo, I was very impressed with the Cancer Treatment Centers of America. If you can't get to one of them, do your research on the internet and find the best facility/doctor you can get to. If your doctor is ignorant about these diets and nutrition in general, don't be surprised. Go to the best health food store you can find; they will not be ignorant about nutrition, and somebody there will know about the ketogenic diet or the rainbow diet. If they don't, get someone there who will be your go-to person and get them to do some research as well. They will be glad they did since this disease is one of the worst plagues of modern society, and they will not be short of interested consumers.

When it comes to vitamins and supplements, use your head and decide on a reasonable number. Research which supplements, vitamins, and herbs are best to treat whatever specific form of the disease you are fighting. You can't spend all day taking vitamins and supplements and drinking herbal teas; you need to be outside in fresh air and sunshine every day and find some joy in the beauty of nature and life itself.[16]

Our first step is getting the best medical care, and the second step is good nutrition. Look at embracing the strict ketogenic twelve-gram disease-starvation diet. However, if you have always been a person with weak willpower about diet and food and cannot alter that self-image, adopt the rainbow diet or something similar. Whichever you choose, eat clean and use the best applicable supplements.

When I was first diagnosed, I got on the computer and made a list of

[16] **Search Phrases: herbs to fight + your diagnosis, vitamins to fight + your diagnosis, supplements to fight + your diagnosis.**

everything known to fight the disease in any of its myriad forms and went on a shopping spree at the health food store. After some time, I concluded that what was best for me was using a good multivitamin plus five to six supplements. I focused on what could improve the immune system or inhibit the reproduction of the bad cells. I was guided by several people at the health food store, which was also the source of some of my best academic information on the terrible properties of sugar.

But let's keep it simple. Adopt the ketogenic diet or an alternative like the rainbow diet, take the appropriate vitamins and supplements, and eat clean. If you eat clean, drink pure, clean water, and breathe deeply, keeping your blood-oxygen level at 98, 99, or 100 percent, you are on a good start to winning the biggest fight of your life. If you don't have the self-discipline to do an extreme twelve-grams-of-carbs-a-day diet, then embrace the rainbow diet or something similar.

## Take the Second Step

Decide on the best diet for you and begin immediately! What exactly is the ketogenic diet? Almost everybody has heard of the Atkins diet. That is a ketogenic diet. You get rid of all sugar, fruit sugar, carbs like breads, and all starches including potatoes. You make your body live off the alternative to sugars—fats and oils. These make ketones. Ketones become your body's alternative energy source instead of sugar—glucose. If you eat tons of leafy greens and get good fats and oils from avocados, macadamia nuts, coconut products such as milk, cooking oil, and yogurt, and unadulterated fish and meats, your body will run clean on ketones.

However, you must be aware that there is a big difference between the Atkins diet to lose weight and the ketogenic twelve-grams-of-carbs-a-day diet to starve cancer. The theory is that if you keep your consumption of total cumulative grams of carbs each day to twelve grams or less, the mutant disease cells will starve to death without glucose. The anecdotal evidence shows the disease either disappears or tumors become benign. This takes work. Each day, it takes a lot of time and work. This diet is almost a full-time job, but it's your life we're talking about. You need accurate charts to depend on; you must eat lots of fresh, organic food. You must plan meals and total all carbs, even the carbs of green leafy vegetables. Chard and lettuce are very low in carbs. You must avoid any hidden sugars, so check your toothpaste. Check everything.

Several people have pointed out to me that I've always been a person of strong will, and not everybody can do such a strict diet—not even to save their own lives. A friend of mine, a young physician I like and respect, estimated that 40 percent of oncology patients would probably be willing to do such a diet. My friend at the CDC thinks it's much lower. I strongly disagree.

First, if you are motivated enough to obtain and read this book, you are already strongly motivated to get well. How many of my readers choose the rainbow diet remains to be seen. I prefer the twelve-gram disease-starvation diet because it is based on crisp clear logic and a Nobel Prize. However, the rainbow diet also has many enthusiastic advocates.

If you try but simply cannot do the twelve-gram disease-starvation diet, then immediately adopt the rainbow diet or something similar. Order the book and follow the diet. Because I didn't study it like I did the twelve-gram disease-starvation diet, I am not an expert on it. After doing my research, I chose the rainbow diet as my fallback diet in the event I couldn't follow the twelve-gram diet. [17]

There may be other low-carb, eat-clean-and-healthy diets that you can use as an alternative. I've read that the rainbow diet has worked successfully for many people, and it made sense to me. If I had not found out how to starve the disease, it is the diet I would have followed. Because I chose the twelve-gram diet and the rainbow as a backup, I am not an expert in all the cancer-fighting diets. I did not go vegan. If your research provides you with a low-carb, clean and nutritious, disease-fighting diet, go for it. Just make sure it is logical and has a track record of success.

## Sugar-Rich Junk Foods, Obesity, and Willpower

I've had heated discussions with a friend who works at the CDC. She won't argue with the Nobel Prize or the reality of my personal results, but she believes most people are too undisciplined and lack the will to eat this way.

---

[17] **Search Phrase: the rainbow diet to beat cancer.**

She hasn't studied this subject, but she thinks most people lack will-power. She thinks most patients would rather eat sugar and suffer and die than be disciplined and eat to live. I strongly disagree. However, many obese and morbidly obese people are addicted to food—just as an alcoholic is to alcohol or a junkie is to heroin. As a society, we greatly underestimate how difficult it is for many people to lose weight, but no one thinks it's easy to quit smoking or go cold turkey. Sugar-rich junk foods are these people's heroin, and they need help and support to beat their addiction.

Obesity seriously increases the chances of getting cancer. If this re-lates to you, get help and support. Don't be proud and think you don't need help. Your addiction to certain types of food is no different than others' cravings for tobacco, alcohol, or heroin. To kick these sugar-rich junk food addictions, you need an iron will, support, and help. Get help in group situations or with counselors and nutritionists. Sugars and car-bohydrates are your enemy; addictions are not easy to defeat, but our society respects all who recognize they have a problem, seek help, take direct action, and overcome their issues.

I think the people who choose to read this book are interested in actively fighting the disease and winning. Willpower and self-discipline are among the most important qualities of the human character; like a muscle, they must be used, and with more use, they become stronger.

If you want to live, you must immediately start avoiding all sugar, foods with added sugar, starches, and breads. If you lack the will and discipline for the extreme twelve-gram diet; begin with the rainbow diet. If your willpower to save your life becomes stronger, you can switch to starving the mutant cells.

Always remember that Stevia is a zero-carb sweetener made from a green leafy plant. It may taste like you're cheating, but you aren't.

Bread was extremely hard for me to give up. There are now bread companies on the internet with greatly reduced carb counts. Do research about taste, texture, etc. There is a bread substitute made from egg whites in the paleo diets, which is known as cloud bread. There are ways to make the twelve-gram disease-starvation diet easier for bread lovers.[18]

If you have not had a difficult life to this point, you must come to

---

[18] **Search Phrase: low-carb bread, cloud bread.**

terms with the fact that life is hard; life is a struggle that sometimes requires sacrifice and the will to fight. At the very least, I urge you to adopt the rainbow diet or something similar. There is no option with sugar; it directly feeds the mutant cells and must go. Use Stevia instead.

If you switch to a ketogenic diet, for two or three days, the transition from glucose to ketones is a major change for your body. I felt like my heart was racing some of the time. If I hadn't known to expect it, I would have been concerned. People experience the change in many different ways so do research so you will know what to expect.

The Macrobiotic Diet

The macrobiotic diet is well known in some circles and its adherents claim it can cure some diseases. I have great respect for Michio Kushi who brought this diet to the US. He wrote over seventy books and was a truly wise and deeply spiritual man. However, rice is a carb. It might not have all the problems of modern genetically modified wheat, but it's still a carb, and carbs feed the mutant cells. (Wheat used to be a chest-high grain, but now the plants are about a foot high. Many people don't want any part of something genetically modified to that extent.)

If you want to live, get on YouTube and listen to Dr. Tom Seyfried, probably the leading expert in this field, and Dominic D'Agostino, the researcher who did the ketogenic study for the navy. You don't have to live on an extreme diet forever—just until you are free and clear. After that, just eat clean and healthy.

# CHAPTER 4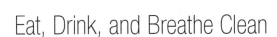

# Eat, Drink, and Breathe Clean

Your immune system is like your body's army and police force. It defends against foreign threats, and it polices and cleans up internal problems. Your immune system is amazing in that it fights the viruses, bacteria, illnesses, and diseases you are exposed to as well as all the natural and artificial environmental toxins your body comes into contact with or takes internally. It does this magnificent job continuously, and we are barely aware of it. Your immune system is always policing the body, looking for mutant and aberrant cells, putting an end to them, cleaning things up, and returning things to normal.

Every so often, for some reason, an immune system is inhibited, overworked, depressed, and not up to its normal efficiency and a mutant, aberrant cell is not immediately killed and disposed of, and it replicates. Then you have the disease. Now you need to jack your immune system into overdrive and clean up the problem that happened when your immune system dropped the ball.

In the 1970s, oncologist O. Carl Simonton began using visualization and meditation to aid the immune system in fighting this disease. You will do this as well. Although he was heavily criticized at the time, it is now a widely accepted practice. You will use diet, your mind, exercise, and deep breathing to jack your immune system into overdrive.[19]

---

[19] **Search Phrases: O. Carl Simonton, boosting your immune system.**

## Clean Food, Pure Water, and Breathing Deeply

If you can get the proper nutrition from clean, unadulterated, unprocessed food, drink a lot of pure filtered water, and breathe deeply on a regular basis, you are freeing your immune system to fight the disease and giving your blood the oxygen it needs.

By doing internet research, you can find out which herbs, vitamins, and supplements will best enhance your immune situation in fighting the specific manifestation of the disease you are dealing with. By selecting and using the best ones, you can rev up your immune system. Clean food and water, the right vitamins and supplements, and a surplus of oxygen allows the immune system to concentrate on attacking mutant cells.

The correct amount of exercise and sleep aids the immune system. Meditation reduces stress, fear, tension, and apprehension, and it enhances well-being. You can use the body-mind-spirit connection to raise your vibes and enhance your immune system throughout the day. If you are fortunate enough to find an integrative oncologist, she or he should be able to guide you through this process.

## Picking the Right Supplements

To fight the golf ball-size adenocarcinoma tumor in my bladder, I bought a wide variety of products and then began narrowing it down to a manageable number of vitamins, herbs, and supplements. If you haven't done so yet, go to your search engine, type in your diagnosis of the specific form of the disease you face, add the plus sign, and use terms such as herbs, vitamins, supplements, and alternative treatments. You will be faced with many choices, some of which have solid scientific research behind them, and some which have been used traditionally in Japan, China, or India for centuries. Just because a major international pharmaceutical company didn't make it does not mean an herb, vitamin, or supplement might not help you substantially. These natural remedies can be strong and must be used intelligently.

I wanted to enhance my immune system and inhibit the growth of the mutant cells. In retrospect, there are other herbs and things I might have added when I learned about them later. I typed in "bladder cancer

+ herbs, vitamins, and supplements," and I ended up using the following to fight the disease:

- astragalus tea and green tea
- age-appropriate multivitamin, vitamin D with omega-3s
- maitake mushroom extract
- grapeseed extract
- curcumin

## The Power of Herbs—Don't Overdo It

To show you the power of herbs, I will once again use my own experience as an example. I liked what I had read about the effects of the astragalus tea, so I drank a lot of it. By that, I mean I drank a whole lot of it. One Friday night, blood showed up in my urine.

Much to my nurse's and my consternation, my urologist—whom I otherwise like and respect—would only see me during office hours and had instructed me to go to the ER if I had a problem after hours. To have no one on call for such a large urological practice seemed lazy and unprofessional to me then and still does. So, I had to go to the ER and see a doctor with no idea about my medical history. After four or five hours of waiting, I finally saw the doctor and told her I was worried about the disease causing so much bleeding. I didn't want to bleed out in my sleep, which might have been highly unlikely, but given the amount of blood in my urine, it did not seem impossible.

After the interviews and some testing, the conclusion was come to that drinking so much of the astragalus tea had irritated my bladder to the point of bleeding. I quit drinking the tea, and the bleeding stopped. Be very aware that the directions and warning concerning herbs, vitamins, and supplements must be adhered to.

## If You Are Stuck with an Unenlightened Doctor

If you are stuck with an unenlightened physician, you must use this book, the internet, and the resources we have suggested to find what is right for you.

This is your fight. You are the general, and your army is your immune system.

The theory is simple. To reinforce your immune system army, bring in all the extra troops, ammunition, and the supplies it needs in its fight against mutations by

- eating clean food,
- drinking pure water,
- breathing deeply three times per day,
- exercising (Western and Eastern styles),
- getting the proper nutrition and supplements,
- getting adequate rest,
- visualizing,
- meditating, and
- using the body-mind-spirit connection properly.

## Building New Good Habits and the Complete Breath

If you do research, you will learn that most forms of meditation reduce stress and anxiety. You know about healing diets. If you are healthy enough, you want at least twenty minutes of cardiovascular exercise every other day as an absolute minimum. It is better if you can walk or run thirty minutes every day and work out with weights at least twice a week, all according to your personal situation. At whatever stage of the disease you begin your self-healing work, try to replace any old unhealthy habits with new healthier ones.

Even if it seems like little of this applies to you because you are in a hospital bed, maybe you can raise that bed's back up and do deep abdominal breathing. One way to develop better breathing habits and raise the oxygen level in your blood is to practice the complete breath several times each day.

The *complete breath* is a way of breathing correctly, like you did as a baby. Basically, you breathe out fully and then fill your lower abdomen, then your chest, and then your clavicle region with air. Like almost any other subject, the instructions on how to do the complete breath can be found on the internet.[20]

## Learn from Your Yoga Teacher or an MD

If you don't take yoga, you can learn it on the net from an MD. Go to your electronic device, get on YouTube, and put in "the complete breath." One of the top YouTube videos is Dr. Surya Pierce showing you how to do it. It is far from the only instructional video on the subject.[21]

One word of warning: if you have been doing an Asian soft martial art like Tai Chi, Chi Kung, or Do-In, do the deep breathing technique you already know.

There are a few differences between some of the Indian and Chinese systems. Do whatever you are more used to, more comfortable with, or like better; both systems will raise the oxygen level in your blood if it is deficient.

## Getting Clean, Healthy Air

Whether you feel strong and healthy and were just diagnosed or are lying in a hospital bed, you can probably do a complete breath self-healing session several times a day.

If you are doing your deep breathing and raising your oxygen level, you will want to maximize your efforts. Unless your chest, rib cage, or lungs are impaired or the air is polluted and poisonous, deep breathing is almost always good for an individual.

But where is the best air with the most oxygen? Again, I will urge you

[20] Search Phrase: the complete breath.
[21] Search Phrases: on YouTube: Dr. Pierce + the complete breath.

to go online. You will find that most oxygen is produced in the ocean. So deep breathing at the beach or out on a boat would seem logical.[22]

One of my spiritual teachers, the late Ruth Stillman—an Esoteric Section-trained Theosophist and one of the thirteen highest-degree Co-Freemason initiates in the world—told me to go and breathe deeply or meditate among pine trees. She said they produced what our etheric bodies needed to be healthy.

Anywhere you are surrounded by green oxygen-producing plants would seem ideal, but in a hospital room, you may have no choice about where you do your complete breaths. Wherever you are, I would think raising your oxygen level can only help. As in all physical practices, you want to ask your doctor or other health care experts to make sure it is appropriate for your situation.

## Getting Clean Air Inside

You will see in your research that specific plants, environments, and eco-systems differ in the amount of oxygen produced. Of interest to anyone confined inside is the work of NASA scientist B. C. Wolverton. He investigated which plants cleaned the air best and produced the most oxygen in the confined areas within space stations. This information can help you increase the oxygen in your living space or hospital room. Again, you must get on the net and do your own research.

According to Wolverton, the plants that clean the air and produce oxygen the best are mother-in-law-tongue, the areca palm, the red-edged dracaena, the Warneck dracaena, and the peace lily. With enough of these plants, you could live in a closed room and still have fresh air. As in all of this, your situation is unique to you. What of this you need to be healthy, only you can decide. But to be in optimum health, I believe our oxygen level should be no lower than 98 percent.[23]

Later in the book we will examine the ACS and CDC recommendations for exercise, you'll be exposed to the benefits of support groups, and you'll learn about life force-building exercises. You have already learned

---

[22] **Search Phrase: oxygen + best places for deep breathing, best places for clean air, how is oxygen produced?**
[23] **Search Phrase: B C Wolverton + clean air.**

the complete breath. If you are healthy enough to exercise, get started. If you are confined to bed, try beginning with three short deep breathing sessions a day and then make them longer.

If you put in the search phrase for "B C Wolverton + clean air" you will find many resources to help you clean the air where you live or in a hospital room.

## Fasting to Fight the Disease

Fasting is an ancient practice that is done for physical and spiritual reasons, and the historical record of it goes back as far as we have religious texts. Spiritual men and women all over the world have always gone to retreat in nature and deprive themselves of food for a time. You may not have the time, ability, or desire to go on a retreat in nature, but you can fast to fight the disease in either of two ways.

There is fasting (no one is saying go without water) for a prolonged period of time such as seventy-two-hours before chemotherapy, which has been shown to reduce the toxicity in the body and make it more tolerable. Although that is documented, three days without food is a long time. I fasted for three days once when I was young and healthy, and it was far from easy. The patient would have to be strong enough to undergo a three-day fast and be very determined.

Fasting has reportedly been helpful for some people when they make the transition from a glucose-fueled body to one depending on ketones. The twelve-gram ketogenic diet works well for some when used in conjunction with daily intermittent fasting, a practice of fasting for sixteen to eighteen hours a day, and consuming meals for a period of six to eight hours.[24]

## Intermittent Fasting

I feel comfortable endorsing a one-day fast when you switch to a ketogenic diet and intermittent fasting used in association with the ketogenic

---

[24] **Search Phrases: fasting to fight cancer, fasting and the ketogenic diet to fight cancer.**

diet. However, I never underwent the poisoning of chemo. For some people, an extended fast may be the proper preparation for chemo.

Some experts advise a daily practice of intermittent fasting in which you limit the time in which you consume food to between six and eight hours. Many practitioners believe this practice makes the ketogenic diet more effective.[25]

Please Google variations on "fasting + fighting cancer," "fasting + your specific form of the disease," and "fasting + the Ketogenic diet to fight cancer." Examine fasting to fight the disease and see how it can make your immune system stronger and more effective. When done intelligently, fasting may be useful ammunition as you fight this disease.

There Is Hope

Mercola.com has an article called "There's Still Hope in Cancer Treatment." Dr. Mercola and research scientist Dr. Dominic D'Agostino talk about the ideal ketogenic diet to defeat the disease.

Dominic D'Agostino suggests the following:

- Low carbs—get most of your carbs from non-starchy vegetables.
- Low protein—about 1 gram of protein per kilogram of body weight (1 gram of protein for every 2.2 pounds).
- Replace your previous glucose producers with the right fats from the following:

  - avocados
  - butter
  - coconut oil
  - macadamia nuts
  - olives

- Get rid of all dairy except for dairy fat (butter and sour cream).

I fasted for twenty-four hours, drinking water and herb teas when I switched to a ketogenic diet and started the twelve-gram disease-starvation diet.

[25] **Search Phrase: intermittent fasting and the ketogenic diet to fight cancer.**

If you fast first, it helps your body make the transition from glucose to ketones. This happens naturally as your body uses up its glucose supply; it begins to transition to using ketones as a fuel naturally.

Some consider fasting an integral part of starting the twelve-gram disease-starvation diet. The transition from glucose to ketones can be a rough one for several days; fasting that first day may be ideal. I also did the intermittent fasting, restricting my eating period to about an eight-hour window.

If you go to the site *collective evolution* on the web, there is an article called "Scientists Discover that Fasting Triggers Stem Cell Regeneration and Helps Fight Cancer." Since fasting is a form of starvation, the body reacts as though it is starving.[26] One thing the body does when starving is to begin recycling old and unhealthy white blood cells.

When you resume consuming healthy food, there is a surge of strong healthy white blood cells.

Fasting can help you fight the disease in many ways:

- A twenty-four-hour fast can help you make the transition from glucose dependence to living on ketones.
- Intermittent fasting helps the immune system work well.
- Fasting beforehand can make chemo less toxic.
- Fasting can strengthen the immune system.

## Avoid Environmental Toxins

The modern world harbors so many dangers. Environmental toxins seem to be everywhere; there are viruses and bacteria. Diseases previously unknown to humans appear, as we face the diseases and plagues of modern life. Google "Environmental Pollutants and the Immune System" and read about two large environmental dangers—aromatic hydrocarbons and phthalates. The first is produced anytime anything burns. This goes from a forest fire to a small campfire, from a wood-burning stove to the charcoal and burn marks on your steak. The second leaches out of

---

[26] **Search Phrases: www.Mercola.com/There's Still Hope in Cancer Treatment and www.collectiveevolution.com/Scientist Discover that Fasting Triggers Stem Cell Regeneration & Helps Fight Cancer.**

hundreds of very common items. The one that affected me would be medical tubing. I had tubing in my body for decades.

Please read the internet article by *Physicians for Social Responsibility* to understand the threats and toxins your immune system faces and normally defeats. Learn what inhibits your immune system—stress, lack of rest, depression, lack of exercise, bad lifestyle (alcohol, drugs, no sleep, etc.), poor nutrition, and polluted air, water, or food. You must avoid as many dangers as possible and do what you can to enhance your immune system.[27]

## Dr. Ray Sahelian

At www.raysahelian.com, a doctor lists the many supplements, herbs, vitamins, diets, foods, and natural and alternative treatments you can use to fight the disease. He lists environmental hazards to avoid. He surprisingly advises you to remove your shoes before entering the house to not bring in environmental toxins and suggests the following:

- filtering your tap water
- using steel, glass, or BPA-free water bottles
- using glass or ceramic and not plastic containers if you microwave
- minimizing use of food grown with pesticides
- minimizing meats raised with antibiotics or growth hormones
- avoiding processed, well done, or charred meats
- reducing medical radiation to a minimum
- avoiding exposure to formaldehyde, benzene, and radon, which is much more common in daily living than most think

Please go to his site and read this in detail. You are already fighting for your life. Give your immune system what it needs to fight with—and don't distract it by making it work unnecessarily to clean up the avoidable toxins you eat, drink, or otherwise come into physical contact with.[28]

---

[27] **Search Phrases: www.psr.org/environmental pollutants and the immune system.**
[28] **Search Phrase: www.raysahelian.com (scroll down and click on cancer).**

## Eat Clean Food, Drink Pure Water

Go to Whole Foods or someplace where you can get organic vegetables in large amounts and organic fruits in much more limited amounts. If you consume meat, it must be free from the hormones and antibiotics found in most of the meat supply. The closer to natural—wild-caught fish, grass-fed, open-pasture, and free-range meat—the better for you. If you live in the modern world, you are exposed to so many toxins. Do your best to avoid them, free up your immune system, and bolster your immune system to do its job and get you healthy.

Pay attention to the toxic dangers listed above. Your water should be filtered, and it is best if you drink it from glass. Don't think you are doing yourself any favors by drinking the supposedly clean commercial water sold in plastic bottles that are available pretty much everywhere.

Anderson Copper was visibly shocked on his TV show when he underwent a test that tells you what's in your body. They found a toxic substance within him that was directly traceable to his plastic water bottle usage. I don't care how pure the water was when it was put into the plastic container, you don't know how much sunshine or heat that bottle was exposed to—or how much leaching has occurred before you drink it, or how many microscopic pieces of plastic went into the bottle during the manufacturing and bottling process.

## Getting Truly Clean Water

Here again, you must do your own research. The easiest way to get clean water is to put a filtration system directly on your faucets, but the ones I found at my local retailers a couple of years ago were a sham. Just because they use the words "pure" or "clean" or "filtered" in their name doesn't mean they do much. I ended up using the GE water pitcher filter system I got at Home Depot, and I immediately substituted using glass jars instead of plastic pitchers. This system renders almost pure water.[29]

When I recently went to Home Depot, there seemed to be a much larger selection of effective products. Be sure to read what they actually

---

29

do. Some of the name-brand water purifiers you see on TV do not really purify the water. Do research and decide what's best for you, but don't get conned by ads on TV. The purer the better; if you can easily afford to purify the water you bathe in as well as drink, it can't hurt.

# CHAPTER 5

# Using Your Mind Positively

## The Difficulty of Changing Belief Systems

Upon diagnosis, many people face an additional dilemma. Many of us have ignored warnings about our jobs, habits, and lifestyles. Once you have been diagnosed, accepting that where you have worked or currently work or live may be a potentially toxic environment—or that your habits, diet, or lifestyle may have contributed to you getting the disease—is not an easy thing for many people in our culture. Suddenly making a transition from the stress-filled, unhealthy average American lifestyle and unhealthy fast-food diet to a healthy lifestyle is not expected to be easy and is certainly not inexpensive. There may also be considerable psychological issues. Changing one's beliefs is extremely difficult for some people, and so is admitting they were wrong about something.

A man who married one of my cousins was a commercial farmer. I think he was just a normal commercial farmer, probably using growth hormones and antibiotics on his animals and pesticides on his crops when he came down with the pancreatic disease that took his life. I don't know any specifics about his farming practices. I'm just using someone like that as an example. If you have worked for decades in commercial agriculture or the chemical, pesticide, printing, furniture, carpeting, or wood businesses, and you have told your family, your employees, or yourself to ignore the warnings from some segments of our culture that your products and practices were unsafe—and you get the disease—then you are faced with the possibility that you were wrong, potentially dead wrong.[30]

It can be very difficult for an individual to face the unpleasant fact that the chemicals or professional practices that you were told—or that you told others were safe—were not safe, and now they have made you ill. What you thought was all medical alarmism or hippy-dippy New Age BS turned out to be true.

It takes an unusually strong human being to

- admit they were wrong,
- admit they may have hurt themselves,
- admit they may have hurt others, and
- change their beliefs and lifestyle.

It is sad to me that a surprisingly high percentage of people would rather die than admit they were wrong, change their belief systems, and adopt a new lifestyle that could save their lives.

My Brother

When my brother (who worked in commercial printing around dangerous chemicals) was diagnosed with leukemia, he absolutely refused to fight the disease in many ways, despite the evidence concerned loved ones presented to him. It almost seemed that because his wife and I were so insistent he could fight in certain ways that he chose not to. For example, he loved cooking over a grill, and he absolutely refused to give up charring the meat, despite the clear evidence that said it was carcinogenic.

He thought, besides medical treatments, he could fight this disease purely with his will and his spirit. He adamantly refused to accept that fighting with will and spirit could include making some disciplined lifestyle changes that his wife and other loved ones were prompting him toward. Sometimes I wonder if we had all left him alone, if he would have eventually come to these conclusions on his own.

When his wife did see any improvement in diet and lifestyle, as soon

---

[30] **Search Phrases: environmental dangers in the home, environmental dangers in the workplace.**

as he was away from her, he would do everything he had been abstaining from. By the time he realized he really did need to fight physically and was willing to change his lifestyle and behavior, it was way too late. It was the last three weeks of his life. You cannot wait to fight this disease; you must begin immediately upon diagnosis to fight with will and determination. Make the needed lifestyle changes with the idea that nothing will stop you from regaining your health.

If you are a person who must change your belief system, behavior, or lifestyle, and you accept it and do it, then I admire you. Sadly, way too many people would rather die than change.

I believe it takes introspection to accomplish this great a change and an internal honesty about oneself that many people lack. If, despite the best of intentions and in accordance with what you were told, you professionally toxically poisoned others and yourself for years and now you are ill, you have many choices to make. Change is incredibly difficult for some people. I wrote this book in the hope my readers will always choose life.

If you are facing major changes and feel a certain amount of guilt, welcome to what many shamanic cultures refer to as "the calling." The calling is a kind of spiritual crisis or awakening that occurs to some when they are seriously injured or ill. It is a calling to change—to live a better, more balanced, and more spiritual life. It may be a calling for someone who has lived a materialistic life to become more spiritual or a calling to return to a spiritual life for someone who has strayed.

## Enhancing Your Immune System

The stress and fast-food diets of many Americans—plus those who smoke, drink too much, or have other bad habits—inhibit an immune system already under constant attack. You can fight stress with exercise and meditation; you can avoid toxins by drinking pure water and eating clean food. Whatever you eat, make sure it is clean. As much as possible, eat unprocessed food. Your fruits and vegetables should be organic—no pesticides, no GMO. Only eat antibiotic-free, free-range, and grass-fed poultry or meat and wild-caught fish. As much as possible, eat and drink free from environmental toxins. Whatever you consume, make it the

cleanest and closest to nature you can get. Get adequate sleep, good nutrition, and raise the oxygen levels in your blood by doing the complete
breath deep-breathing exercise three times a day to aid your immune
system in fighting internal threats.

The theory here is that your immune system is your primary internal self-healing mechanism. You want to do things that enhance your
immune system and quit doing things that inhibit your immune system
so your immunity army is not hindered by you and the things you do in
small daily skirmishes and is left unencumbered and free to fight the real
war and defeat the real enemy—the disease.

You want to cheer your army on—not sabotage it. As far as I'm concerned, giving aid to your enemy in a time of war is treason. If you have
this disease, you are under attack. Fight to win—and I have three small
tricks to help.

## Three Tricks for Better Health

In the body-mind-spirit approach to becoming free and clear, I have three
keys I've learned from decades in a wheelchair. The first is gut health.
Some claim 70 percent of your immune system is in your gut. Many antibiotics and common medicines wipe out the flora of your intestines. You
must reseed your gut with probiotics. Again, the internet will be full of
info and ads. Ask your health food store folks which product is best for
you and use the right probiotics to reseed your gut.[31]

The second is a clean mouth: healthy and clean gums, teeth, and
tongue. A gum infection can easily move into your bloodstream, leading
to serious problems. If you are reading this book, I bet you've got enough
problems and don't need any more. Keeping a clean mouth is part of a
good defense strategy. Get an electric toothbrush, use good, natural, no-
sugar toothpaste, and gargle with salt water. (If you prefer commercial
products, don't gargle with anything containing food coloring.) Brush
your teeth so long at least once a day that it feels to your tongue as though
you just went to the dentist. Read a book, watch TV, whatever, and just

---

[31] **Search Phrase: percent of immune system in gut.**

brush your teeth, gums, tongue, everywhere in your mouth to get it completely clean. Then gargle with salt water.

The last good health tip is something I learned when I had a broken femur that wasn't healing. I had six six-inch screws on the inside/outside of my left leg and a brace called a fixator. Bathing was difficult. I found out you don't want your physical health problems to spill over into psychological issues.

You must bathe and do your personal hygiene as though you were going out in public every day. Do not skip bathing; don't lie around in a robe; or skip combing your hair, washing your face, or shaving. Not grooming is simply inviting depression to the party. In the mystical tradition, we think bathing with intent can work the body-mind-spirit connection to aid mental and physical well-being, so bathe daily, groom daily, dress and look good.

If you eat clean food, drink pure water, breathe deeply, get exercise, sleep well, calm your mind, and defeat stress, it enhances your immune system and leaves it free to fight your real problem at full strength.

Modern medicine is developing more targeted therapies, and surgeries can remove diseased organs or tissue. There are always exceptions, but in the most simple and general terms, much of what they do is to help your own immune system contain and destroy the disease. In the end, your immune system will lose or win this fight. By living clean and enhancing your immune system, you are giving it the best chance to win. If you doubt the basic premise, go to your computer, type in "immune system + kills cancer," and you will see that the immune system is the key to the body fighting and defeating this disease—now and in the future.[32]

Once you are clean and well-nourished inside—cheering on and enhancing your immune system—you will train and use your mind to aid your body. In the mystical tradition, we have worked the body-mind-spirit combination for thousands of years, using the three aspects of a human. Mystics have long worked with what various schools of thought call the subconscious, the conscious, and the superconscious or the id, ego, and superego, or the low self, middle self, and high self. Although different fields of modern psychology do not always agree on the definitions of these terms, in this book, I use terms the average reader will understand.

[32] **Search Phrase: immune system + kills cancer cells.**

I use the terms *conscious, subconscious, and superconscious* and equate them to the ego, id, and superego and to the middle self, low self, and high self.

In the 1970s O. Carl Simonton began using some of the visualization techniques we will use. He was viciously attacked by his fellow doctors for practices that are now standard. I'm sure this book will be called voodoo medicine by the haters just like his was. This same kind of animosity is something you may face from conventional doctors and oncologists— so be prepared. If you are straddled with such a hater, just don't tell him what you are doing. Just do it, and after you have great results, educate him if possible.

Find the best modern medicine fit for your personal situation, decide on the best diet for you, learn how to eat and drink clean, and breathe deeply at least three times a day. Now it is time to learn the correct use of the mind to stimulate your immune system and self-healing mechanisms.

## Beginning the Holistic Battle

By now, you

- have been diagnosed,
- have chosen what you want from the best of modern medicine,
- have decided on a treatment plan you agree with,
- are drinking pure water and eating clean—either the ketogenic or rainbow diet,
- have started breathing deeply three times a day, and
- have started taking the appropriate vitamins and supplements.

It's time to fully use the mind. It's time to unite body, mind, and spirit to fight and win the biggest fight of your life. It's time for visualization, affirmation, and understanding the power of suggestion in human health and human behavior. It is time to activate your body, mind, and spirit to win this fight.

Your spiritual beliefs are personal. However, many studies have shown people who pray, people of faith generally, have better medical results than those not so inclined. However, even if you are a person without faith, you can still use visualization, affirmation, and positive suggestion.

## Uniting Body, Mind, and Spirit in One Purpose

In the West, we know what Jesus taught: as a man believes in his heart, so he is. One way to interpret that is as a man believes (in his conscious mind) and in his heart (his subconscious mind), so he is. Where there is agreement in the conscious and subconscious, there is manifestation.

I would take this farther. If the three aspects of a human being can work together, if the low self - id - subconscious, and the middle self - ego – conscious mind, and the higher self – superego - superconscious mind all work together in agreement, there will be positive manifestation and powerful results.

The tools to unite body, mind, and spirit are as follows:

- visualization
- affirmation
- meditation
- prayer (for believers)
- deep breathing, stretching, and cardiovascular exercise
- basic vibe raising

## Patients with the Best Results

When I first went to the Mayo Clinic in Jacksonville years before my diagnosis, I was fighting early onset osteoporosis and osteomyelitis. I had broken both femurs within a year and had a resistant infection in my broken left femur that wouldn't heal. The doctor asked me what I wanted. I told her I had been a national champion fencer, a Paralympic athlete, and a black belt martial artist who had been fighting full-contact karate against able-bodied opponents at the dojo, but all that was gone. I wanted my life back. I told her I was a motivated patient, that I visualized, prayed, did Tai Chi, Qi Gong, and yoga, and practiced positive thinking.

She said, "Good. You're the kind of patient who has the best results."

I asked her how long it would take for me to get my life back, and her response was two years; two and a half years later, I had my life back.

After my personal disaster at MD Anderson, it was only natural that I would turn back to Mayo. I did examine a local option. There was a doctor working near where I live at Emory University Hospital who was famous for treating the bladder. A good example of just how broken our medical system can be is Emory Hospital, where I was born. It is a nationally renowned hospital, yet I talked on the phone with them for weeks getting the runaround. Finally, I found out part of their problem. As a teaching hospital, each head of a department is like a god unto themselves. One department would accept my insurance, but another department we would need wouldn't. Is that really any way to run a major hospital? After a couple of weeks of bureaucratic nonsense, I gave up on Emory.

I called the orthopedic department at Mayo and left a message for Dr. Mary O'Connor. In the entire ordeal, she was the only medical professional who showed me any real emotion at all. I called her secretary on a Friday to explain my situation, and Dr. O'Connor left a message on my answering machine that afternoon. She was fighting back tears as she said how sorry she was to hear the news about the disease and that I could expect a message by Wednesday about which doctor I should see there. My phone rang first thing Monday morning with the name Dr. Paul Young.

When I went to Mayo, things moved incredibly quickly. Finally, people understood the urgency I felt. So far, all the mutant cells had stayed put in my bladder. However, I'd been given some dire warnings over the years, and I wanted my treatment to move quickly. They did as well.

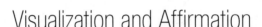

# CHAPTER 6

# Visualization and Affirmation

We've gone over steps 1 and 2 of my eight-point plan, deciding what treatments you want from the best modern medical care available, adopting the best clean and healthy diet and lifestyle, and daily deep breathing. Next let's look at your mental tools: visualization, affirmation, meditation, and prayer. We'll also look at exercise: Western exercises such as walking, cardiovascular work-outs, and weight training and Eastern deep-breathing exercises like yoga, Tai Chi, and Chi Kung.

We've already touched on raising vibes; we'll expand on that as well. Out of these many techniques, let's begin with visualization. Some would say it is the most powerful tool in your arsenal, and others would strongly argue for diet. It is the "you are what you eat" school of thought versus the "if you can see it, visualize it, you can achieve it" school of thought. Both are powerful tools for self-healing and should be combined.

I am yet to meet a human who says they have no imagination and never daydream. Visualization is just the normal human act of using one's imagination, but it can be improved, disciplined, and refined to become a creative force within the human psyche. You can find many authors and experts on the power of the mind who consider visualization an incredibly powerful tool that is readily available to you; it is a tool of the mind that has been used for thousands of years.[33]

---

[33] **Search Phrase: visualization + fighting cancer.**

## Visualization Made Easy

In the mystical tradition we are told that thousands of years ago, in the classical Greek and Roman cultures, visualization was one of the tools the initiates of the mystery schools would use to shape their lives and their world. In modern terms, you use visualization to reprogram your biocomputer. You will train your conscious mind to utilize and refine your imagination to reprogram your subconscious mind and your superconscious mind to do everything possible to mobilize your internal self-healing mechanisms to bring you to a state of health.

You use visualization to reprogram your biocomputer to be a healthy, free, and clear (of all disease) human. You use your imagination to see yourself healthy and well at the end of this journey. You do this by directing and starring in your own quick video clip of the imagination.

Decide on a very short scene, exactly as if you are writing and directing a short movie.

You might imagine a scene where your doctor is telling you that all the tests show you are now well and healthy. You might imagine a scene where you are celebrating your wellness with your spouse, or maybe a scene telling your best friend you are free and clear. Create a short movie scene in your imagination in which you can easily see yourself, that tells the story of you achieving your health. Imagine a scene that comes to you easily—one you can believe in. It would be best if, somewhere in your movie scene, you say some phrase conveying that you are healthy and well, well and whole, or free and clear.

Refine this image of the doctor telling you that all the tests show you are well or celebrating that you are free and clear, whatever you choose. Add as many senses as you can into this blueprint for what you desire. Be aware of the lighting, the way your body feels, how the room feels, and any sounds or smells you might associate with that place. Add as many of your five senses as possible into your imagining of the short scene. I imagined reporting back to my favorite doctor that all the tests showed I was free and clear and that I was perfectly healthy, well, and whole.

At first develop your short film in a relaxed state. Get relaxed and imagine it bit by bit, word by word. Once you have written and directed your movie in your mind, watch it, be it, and live it in your imagination.

Once you know your short film by heart, you can relax and add conscious, relaxed deep breathing as you watch it and live it.

Regaining your health can be, should be, and really must be a full-time job. Visualization is a major component of that job.

We are giving you a working plan with many tasks:

- finding the best modern medicine available
- deciding on a plan of treatment you agree with
- eating clean food, drinking pure water, and breathing deeply
- getting on the ketogenic diet to starve mutant cells
- or utilizing the rainbow diet or something similar
- using visualization, affirmations, meditation, and prayer
- exercising using Western cardiovascular and weight training exercises
- and Eastern deep breathing, stretching, life force building exercises
- raising your vibes and changing your frequency to the most positive and healthiest you can every day

If you can do your visualization while deep breathing or doing deep breathing exercises like Qi Gong, that is wonderful. The same thing with affirmation, it is more powerful combined with relaxed deep breathing and deep-breathing exercises.

The more you can combine these techniques, the more time you save in your busy day. And if done correctly, the more powerful they can be in self-healing.

## Affirmation and Self-Suggestion

If all of this is new to you, or if you are an agnostic or atheist with little interest or belief in the spiritual, maybe you are familiar with the TV series that ran for many years. In *The Mentalist,* the main character worked as a consultant with law enforcement despite his colorful background as a sideshow carnie fake psychic. He used suggestion, hypnosis, and other tools of the mind to read people, elicit confessions, and otherwise solve crimes. You will be using the same tools except you won't be solving crimes—you'll be mobilizing your internal self-healing mechanisms.[34]

Your personal outlook may be that of an agnostic or atheist, and you may feel all religion is just human imagination and that my personal mysticism is silly. That doesn't bother me at all. I run into this in my own family. Your lack of belief in the supernatural doesn't mean you shouldn't use all the tools of modern psychology available to you. To not use the tools recognized and accepted in modern psychology to boost your immune system and mobilize your internal self-healing mechanisms seems stupid and lazy to me.

As an agnostic or atheist, you can at least admit to the reality of a conscious and subconscious mind. Most of you will even admit to a human conscience, which leads to Freud's superego and to the concept of the superconscious. If you will go this far, there is one very powerful form of visualization/prayer available. Even if you will not agree to the superconscious, you can still use visualization, affirmation, and the principles of self-suggestion to mobilize the potent forces of your own internal self-healing mechanisms to boost your immune system and move you toward health and well-being.

## The Power of Affirmations

Although this is a body-mind-spirit approach to self-healing, if you just do the body and mind part right, you can work this system successfully. If detection, treatment, and the twelve-gram starvation diet are begun early enough, and patients do these things every day correctly, earnestly, with self-discipline, their success rate will be significantly higher than those who passively take treatment and eat normal sugar-rich diets. I have no doubt the anecdotal evidence of my readers will pile up quickly.

The use of affirmation may be considered by some as a kind of self-hypnosis. So what? If it is effective, who cares what it is called? Years ago, I took a twenty-hour course in clinical hypnosis and came away in absolute awe of the power of the subconscious mind. To begin practicing your affirmations, you may just relax in front of a mirror, take a few

---

[34] **Search Phrase: affirmation + defeating cancer.**

relaxed deep breaths, and say *your version* of something like one or two of the following:

- I have a strong and powerful immune system - an all-conquering immune system.
- I am perfectly healthy, well, and whole.
- I am free and clear, perfectly healthy, well and whole.
- I am now, and I am become perfectly healthy, well, and whole.
- I am healthy, free and clear.

Although these statements may not actually describe your current condition, you are reprogramming your body-mind to be healthy, well, free, and clear. You must imagine positively and in the present tense what you want to be your physical reality in the near future.

## Program Only Positives—Never Negatives

It is probably best if you make up your own personal affirmations. Any statement that feels natural for you to say and affirms your reclaimed health and well-being will work. As you say these things out loud, feel them and believe them internally.

One of the most important things taught in that hypnosis class was that the subconscious is like a pet or a child and doesn't necessarily understand much in a sentence except the main words; therefore, use positive suggestions, and never use a negative or double negative.

If your suggestion is in negative terms, you are probably instructing/ programming your subconscious to work against you. One of the worst suggestions you can make to yourself, even with the best of intentions, is this: I hope this cancer isn't too bad. I hope it doesn't spread.

Your subconscious may only get three words from that—the name of the disease, the word *bad*, and the word *spread*.

And your subconscious and your biocomputer just got programmed by you to work against you in the worst possible way. You are basically telling yourself you are not choosing life.

- Make all your affirmations and self-suggestions as positive as possible!
- I am healthy, free and clear, well and whole!
- I have a strong and powerful all-conquering immune system!

As in your visualizations, the suggestions you are making to yourself must be for good, achievable goals, couched in the most positive words available.

Remember that time is something for the conscious mind; the goals with which you reprogram your subconscious mind must be stated in the present. You are programming your biocomputer with what you want to be real in your present tense. Also remember there is always a cure rate, and that unexplained spontaneous remissions do occur, at all stages, especially with this disease. You are doing this work so that you are a person who is healed. Whether the cure rate is 95 percent, 80 percent, 60 percent, 30 percent or 5 percent, be determined to be in that group; be resolute that you will obtain a free and clear state and remain healthy.

Suggest to yourself with powerful affirmation your version of "I am now, and I am become perfectly healthy, well, and whole. I have a strong and powerful, an all-conquering immune system."

In your daily conversations, your goal is to be "free and clear." Don't use the phrase "cancer-free." You should never even use the name of the disease except when medically necessary. Don't look stupid at the doctor's office; use the correct medical terminology in that environment. However, never use the name of the disease in your affirmations or self-suggestions. I wouldn't use the *m* word either—the word equivalent for "spreading."

## Avoid Negativity—Be Positive

If you need to explain things to family or friends, try to remain positive and use positive words. When asked how I was doing, I would say that my body seemed to be fighting it well, that the tests showed that all the mutant cells were staying put, and that I was exercising and eating healthy. I tried to answer their questions, but I kept my thoughts and their thoughts as positive as possible. [35]

I had one brother who seemed to me to be very negative in his questioning. I had to avoid talking to him or cut all conversations short. He meant well, his intentions were good, but he was so relentlessly negative. It was exasperating. When I tried to explain exactly how I felt, he didn't understand and was totally oblivious to what I was saying. No matter what I said, he was determined not to hear or understand my complaints about how negative his relentless questioning was. I felt like a criminal being grilled by the bad cop in a movie.

You just do the best you can, stay positive, talk positive, and if you must, avoid the negative people in your life. Tell yourself you have a strong and powerful immune system as you feed and empower your immune system with oxygen from deep breathing and healthy foods and supplements. Use your mind to rev up your immune system and throw it into overdrive.

## Begin Combining Your Techniques

We have gone over the basics of visualization and affirmation. Once you feel comfortable with both techniques for reprogramming your subconscious, you can save precious time by combining them.

Have a short statement of your regained health in your visualization. While deep breathing, in a relaxed state, whisper or say your affirmation when you reach that part of your film. Say, "I'm free and clear. I'm incredibly healthy."

Incorporate your affirmations into your visualization. Picture yourself with a friend or loved one in your visualization and say, "I am healthy, free, and clear." You can think, whisper, or say the actual words out loud.

In a coming section, we will review many of the Eastern deep-breathing and stretching exercise systems. You can decide which of the Eastern deep-breathing stretching system you will enjoy most from:

---

[35] **Search Phrase: positive attitude + fighting cancer.**

- yoga
- Qi Gong (there are various spellings)
- medical Qi Gong
- Tai Chi
- Do-in, the self-healing exercise system of Michio Kushi

You may incorporate your visualization/affirmation with many of the repetitive movements found in such systems.[36]

## Embrace the Simplicity

The reader may wonder if there shouldn't be more to this part of my program than these few pages. If these are such powerful tools to reprogram the human biocomputer, shouldn't there be more than these few pages? The short answer is no.

It really is this simple. Just imagine the scene, put all your senses into it, put your affirmation in, and imagine the joy you feel being free and clear, healthy, and well. Just relax and breathe fully and deeply. Through repetition, you reprogram your biocomputer. The power of these techniques comes from the force of your will and the power of repetition.

You can start with your affirmations in front of the mirror. With the body relaxed, breathe deeply. When you say it, imagine the joy you feel being well and past all this.

Visualization is nothing more than the willful and disciplined refining of your imagination. One of my teachers taught a technique in which you try to imagine a theater screen between your eyes and see yourself healed on that screen. Basically, you watch your visualization movie on your third-eye flat-screen. I just tell people to use their imagination naturally, create a short movie, and as you watch it, feel it, say it, try to include as many of your senses in it as you can, especially feel the joy of being well and moving past this struggle.

The power of the technique comes from your will, your intention, your expectation, and the simple power of repetition in reprogramming

---

[36] **Search Phrases: yoga, Qi Gong, Medical Qi Gong, Tai Chi, Michio Kushi.**

your biocomputer. The technique is simple and powerful, and you must do it every day without fail.

But a word of warning: Never visualize and drive! Although we take driving for granted and allow almost anyone to drive in this country, every time you get behind the wheel, you are responsible fo your safety, your passengers' safety, and other drivers and pedestrians.

Visualization done correctly involves too much of your brain; you cannot visualize and operate a car safely. Driving is a huge responsibility—so pay attention while driving.

Don't be put off by the simplicity of these techniques. The power comes from you, your will, and the power of repetition to program the human biocomputer, allowing you to tap into the vast power of the human mind.

# CHAPTER 7

# Causation, Your Spiritual Beliefs, and the "Why Me?" Question

## Higher Power and Spiritual Belief Systems

Most people express a belief in a higher power, although the conceptions of that higher power vary widely. In the United States, it is consistently over 90 percent who believe, with 50 percent of the population praying at least once a day. Surprisingly, 20 percent of self-described atheists had belief in a higher power of some sort—just not the God described in conventional religions.

One of my spiritual teachers—the woman I called by the Native American title of respect, Grandmother Evelyn Eaton was part Indian like myself and was a prolific and highly respected author, poet, and academic. During her time, Warner Brothers purchased her book *Silently My Captain Waits*, and she was published repeatedly by the best magazines. She was a best-selling author who wrote twenty-six books, and three were about her journey into shamanism. You can Google her and find she still has books in print and being reprinted.[37]

Grandmother Eve once told me something I found profound. She told me we had all come from the Great Spirit and were each created with an individual divine spark from and of the Creator. She taught me once we have been created, we have an immortal divine spark and spirit, and as we grow and evolve, we become cocreators with the Great Spirit. We are

---

[37] **Search Phrase: Evelyn Eaton.**

not eventually absorbed by the oneness as taught in some philosophies, but we continue growing and evolving as immortal divine beings.

## Why Me?

Grandmother Eve once told me that we had all come from the Great Spirit, and there are as many paths back to the Great Spirit as there are people. It was like highways, surface roads, dirt roads, trails, and footpaths. Most people took the superhighways of the major religions, some took the smaller surface streets of the lesser known religions and sects, and others took their own individual paths.

Grandmother Eve taught all these paths led back to the Great Spirit and were all equally valuable to the person who traveled them. The agnostic or atheist reader may not be interested in how belief systems, religious practices, and faith can affect the self-healing process, but this can be highly important for many readers.

Many readers will naturally ask, "Why me? Why did I get this disease at this time in my life? What caused it?" Depending on the reader, they may look to various levels of causation.

The agnostic or atheist will look only to physical causation. Was it the pollution of our water and air, the use of dangerous insecticides and fertilizers polluting the food supply, the use of antibiotics and growth hormones in agribusiness, the use of preservatives in processed food, prolonged exposure to toxins in the home and workplace, and personal pollution? Did they drink hard liquor, use processed tobacco, or have an unhealthy lifestyle?

Another important question is that of exposure for long periods of time to unhealthy levels of electromagnetic radiation. When a friend of mine asked the oncologist just what caused the mutated cells forming the tumors in his wife's brain, the oncologist asked if she slept with her head close to a radio alarm clock. That may give many people pause to consider where their radio alarm clock is. How many inches or feet is it from their heads?

This disease in all its myriad forms is a plague of our modern society. The more we poison our food, our air, our water, and our bodies with processed food, tobacco, and hard liquor, the more we eat fast food, added sugar, processed everything, the more we live high-stress lives without adequate sleep, the more likely disease is. The more our airways are filled with ever-increasing electromagnetic pollution, the more we carry cell phones on our belts or touching our heads, the more we sleep next to radio alarm clocks, the more tumors will occur.

Investigate for yourself the dangers of EMF (electromagnetic fields) and EMR (electromagnetic radiation). Investigate the dangers of EMR, examine the dangers in your environment, and see what you can do to lessen your exposure. Move your alarm a few feet away and decide if you want the commercially available cell phone and laptop shields.[38]

Although doctors and scientists can give much more complex explanations, in an overall way, the occurrence of this disease can be broken down into general and simple terms. Mutant cells occur every day in our bodies, and our immune system kills them. This happens every day, over and over. Our immune system kicks mutant cell butt. This disease occurs when the immune system is too inhibited to do its job to hunt and kill mutant cells. And the mutant cells multiply.

These mutant cells, as shown in the Warburg's 1931 Nobel Prize work, are different from normal cells in that they consume sugar much faster and may replicate quicker than normal cells. Why did it happen? Was your immune system overworked dealing with all the pollution and poisons going into your body? Were you overworked, overstressed, not getting enough sleep, or depressed?

Dr. Norman Shealy pointed out a clear statistical correlation between chronic depression and cancer. He was not claiming that depression causes the disease; he was just pointing out the numbers.[39]

## Dealing with Depression

I am no scientist, but if depression inhibits the immune system, it certainly isn't helping you to be healthy. Things may also go in the other order; not that depression weakened the immune system, which may

---

[38] Search Phrases: dangers of radio alarm clocks, danger + electromagnetic pollution, danger + EMR, EMF.

[39] Search Phrases: chronic depression + higher cancer risk, chronic depression + weakened immunity, Dr. Norman Shealy.

have contributed to the patient contracting the disease, but that patients often get depressed because of the disease. Having a serious disease and facing death could bring depression on in almost anyone.

You can fight this tendency by getting good modern medical help, taking control of your treatment plan, changing your diet, and using your mind and body to work for you. The more you use these techniques, fill your day with self-healing activities, and eat healthy, the less likely you are to be depressed.

Dr. O. Carl Simonton was using techniques borrowed from the mystical tradition—meditation and visualization—and he was attacked by the close-minded haters in the medical community. He wrote two books on the self-healing process, and you can find him on YouTube, Google, Wikipedia, etc. If you would rather get your techniques from a medical doctor than someone who studied a continuous shamanic tradition that is thirty thousand years old, get his books and use his techniques. You may also want to investigate the Simonton Cancer Center.[40]

## Causation and the Spiritual Aspect

Some people may accept a purely physical explanation for how they got the disease and others look to a more spiritual or metaphysical source. It is natural to wonder why out of everybody in this city, state, nation, why did I get this disease at this time in my life?

Jesus taught as a man sows, so shall he reap. In India, China, and Japan, they accept the concept of karma. In the mystical tradition, we are taught Newton's laws apply to nonphysical levels of causation as well, that the concepts of cause and effect, and of action and reaction are metaphysical as well as physical.

A mystic may believe he contracted a physical disease that had physical causes but that he succumbed to the disease at this point and time because of causes from this lifetime or a past lifetime. Some mystics think that their own divine spirit selected before incarnation the challenges that the soul-mind-body must face and overcome in that lifetime.

---

[40] **Search Phrases: O. Carl Simonton, simontoncenter.com, and his books** ***Getting Well Again, The Healing Journey.***

To such a mystic, the divine spirit does not choose unwisely. This challenge is an opportunity for growth and spiritual evolution. It is the result of causes and effects, but it was selected by the divine spirit—the higher self—ahead of time. It occurred at this moment in time for a reason—as an opportunity for spiritual growth.

## The Whole Armor of God

A Christian may think the disease is a test sent by the Lord or by his dark counterpart. Whoever they think might be the spiritual source, it is still an opportunity to embrace and grow closer to God, to reaffirm their faith, to put on the whole armor of God, and fight the good fight to regain their health.

I was taught by Grandmother Eve and other spiritual teachers that Christians may want to arm themselves using imagination combined with prayer drawing from Ephesians 6:10–18. They can put on the whole armor of God.[41]

- Your loins are girted with the truth.
- You put on the breastplate of righteousness.
- Your feet are shod with the gospels of peace.
- You take up the shield of faith.
- You wear upon your head the helmet of salvation.
- You take up the sword of spirit, which is the Word of God.

Thus armed, you are invincible to any force of darkness. It is the only such spiritual protection prayer in the entire Holy Bible. If you are a Christian, you might want to put on the whole armor of God on a daily basis. You can put *whole armor of God* into your search engine and find many entries.

## Causation and Belief Systems

Grandmother Eve talked about the journey back home to the Great Spirit. Grandmother Eve believed in reincarnation, so she saw this path back to

---

[41] **Search Phrase: Whole Armor of God.**

the Great Spirit as a passage of many, many lifetimes. Speaking in general, in the classical mystery school traditions of Greece and Rome, and in the mystical tradition around the world, reincarnation is an accepted part of the belief systems.

I would like the reader to understand the spiritual worldview of my teachers, but I'm not trying to change anyone's outlook. This self-healing system will work in a way not affected by your belief or disbelief in an afterlife. At the same time, most people in the United States don't believe in reincarnation and are not well educated on the concept.

Although the esoteric Christians can point out many seeming references to the concept of people living more than once in the scriptures, most current Christian leaders in the West choose to interpret their scriptures as indicating that human life is a one-time manifestation. In the Bible it is asked if John the Baptist was Elijah come back—or was Jesus Elijah returned? If the concept of reincarnation was unknown to the people of that time, why would the concept of the prophets returning have been included in both Old and New Testament prophecy scriptures?

Some argue the concept of reincarnation was so widely accepted by the people of that time that it was understood, taken for granted, and inferred repeatedly in the scriptures. Examples of many early church leaders who accepted reincarnation as part of Christianity may indicate that reincarnation was a standard aspect of Christianity until the AD 600s.[42]

The idea is put forward in the mystical tradition that the ruler of the Roman Empire, Justinian outlawed belief in reincarnation in AD 553 because he thought the population was too hard to control believing in many lives; that the one-life heaven-or-hell scenario led to a better-behaved populace due to fear.

What is clear historically is that he did this in a council opposed by the pope and thought to have sparse spiritual authority. Put into your search engine "Justinian + outlaw reincarnation" if you want a fuller picture. Until that point, reincarnation was accepted by many prominent proponents of Christianity.[43]

---

[42] **Search Phrases: St. Augustine, St. Jerome, and Origen (founding fathers of the early church and believers in reincarnation).**
[43] **Search Phrases: mystical tradition + reincarnation, Justinian outlawed reincarnation.**

The reason I have digressed about reincarnation is that we are dealing with the subjects of causality and mortality—the "why me, what was the cause of the disease, why did this happen to me" questions. The agnostic or atheist, the one-life heaven-or-hell believer, the fundamentalist, and the advocate of reincarnation may all approach these questions differently.

In the mystical traditions I was exposed to, your divine spirit, your higher self, chooses before incarnation, guided by the law of cause and effect, what challenges you face during any lifetime. This gives the mystic the feeling—what the heck, my divine spirit chose this challenge for my soul-mind-body to face at this moment in my life—so I better get to facing it. The mystic may also see it as a calling to become a better person, live a more spiritual life, or become a healer. The conventional Christian may also look at this as a calling back to a better life, a calling back to God, or a calling to receive one of the gifts of the Holy Spirit.

Plato, Pythagoras, and many early church figures such as Origen all believed the events of this life were put in motion by previous lives. The mystical tradition teaches that the divine spirit of the individual chooses those challenges presented by the laws of cause and effect before incarnation to teach the evolving soul of the individual certain spiritual lessons.

The one-way believer or fundamentalist Christian may believe the disease comes from the Lord teaching them a lesson or calling them back to a spiritual life—or it may be understood to be an attack by evil. In many spiritual traditions, the physical world, including the human body, are the battleground where the war between good and evil is fought. In other traditions, becoming unhealthy is simply an imbalance that needs to be corrected.

While I was training with Grandmother Eve and Grandfather Raymond, many of our patients at the sweat lodge had gone to see doctors, and their prognosis was not good. Many patients came to a shamanic healer as an absolute last resort. Grandfather Raymond, the highly respected Northern Paiute shaman, told me once in a surprising moment during my personal instruction that my most important job as a healer was to help the person find meaning and purpose in their journey. Whether they regained their health or passed on into the spiritual realm,

I must make sure their journey had meaning. Considering everything a shaman might do to help a patient, it was an important statement.

Whether a person believes in only one life, in reincarnation's many lives, or is an agnostic or atheist, a person's life and the fight for health should have meaning and purpose.

For those curious about reincarnation, interesting books have been written, and academic research is being carried out concerning the phenomenon of children who seem to have accurate memories of a past life. Academic research was done at Duke University and the School of Medicine at the University of Virginia concerning this recurrent and widespread phenomenon.[44]

This concept of reincarnation is not part of implementing this self-healing system, and I don't want the Evangelical or one-way reader to think I'm crazy or anti-Christian and put this book down. Again, if this concept of biblical reincarnation is new to you, look it up on Google or use any good search engine for a lively debate. There are many books about reincarnation as the missing or overlooked element of Christianity. Also be aware that that more people around the world believe in reincarnation than the one-life heaven-or-hell concept.

The agnostic or atheist, as well as many believers, look to a scientific explanation and a specific physical cause of the illness. The pollution of air, water, and food, industrial pollution, toxic workplaces, and the toxic elements of housing, furniture, carpeting, are all likely contributors, and so are processed tobacco, hard liquor, and bad lifestyles. Main contributors can be benzene, radon, and formaldehyde. In fact, every reader should go to their computer and research the things people should avoid to prevent this disease. You should certainly avoid them now if you are already fighting it.[45]

Whether you believe in a purely physical cause, a physical cause manipulated by spiritual forces, whether you think you are a casualty in an ongoing spiritual war between good and evil, or just feel out of balance and harmony, the challenge you face now is to fight for your health. This challenge is inescapable. Whatever your belief system may

[44] **Search Phrases: Duke + reincarnation + Rhine; U of VA med school + reincarnation.**
[45] **Search Phrase: things to avoid + prevent cancer.**

be, overcoming this challenge—becoming free and clear and healthy—may be the most empowering thing you've ever done. Imagine the joy you will feel in this victory. Feel it in your visualization and affirmations, work hard, and do everything you can to make that joy your reality.

## CHAPTER 8 ▌▌▌▌▌

# Prayer and Meditation

Whatever religious beliefs you have, whether you are a fundamentalists/ literalist of any major religion, whether you are conservative or liberal, whether you believe in one-life heaven or hell or believe in many lives, your religion encourages you to pray for others and yourself. In whatever manner you may pray, pray for the health and well-being of others first and then pray for yourself.

Many experts think it is better to try to do this in the same place each day, giving you the best-possible conditions in which to pray. In my humble opinion, prayer is a simple praising, thanking, or asking for help.

Whenever the subconscious mind is involved, as in the act of prayer, ask for things in the most positive words, in the present tense. One technique is to simply give thanks for someone being healthy while you visualize them being healthy; do that for everyone you pray for. Don't get too carried away. I say my general prayers for the well-being of my family and friends and thanks for my teachers and all spiritual help, and I have a serious prayer list with a maximum of eight people. Whatever your religion, you can probably do something similar. A one-way Christian may give thanks to Jesus or the Holy Spirit seeing their loved ones well and whole, feeling all the joy and happiness that healing brings. Whatever your religion, pray with positive images and words, see the people well, and give thanks for their recovery. The net is full of information on the healing power of prayer.[46]

Someone without such specific religious beliefs might just send these

---

[46] **Search Phrase: the healing power of prayer.**

prayer-like images of health and joy to *the source energy*. A New Age but nonreligious person might like the techniques of Christine Sheldon and her talks on YouTube such as "How to Raise Your Frequency to Change your Life." She teaches a nonreligious form of meditation/prayer that may be effective for those without specific religious affiliation.[47]

Prayer for others while you are fighting a disease is not a personal willing—and *never* attempt to send forth your own psychic energy. You are simply asking for someone to be healthy and putting forward a positive mental image of what you are asking for. Some people light candles, incense, sage, or a combination of these. A Native American may pray with a Sacred Pipe. Many readers will already have a personal altar and use the traditional prayers of their culture and religion. Whatever way you do these things, imagine the desired successful results in the present tense and give joyful thanks for their healing as though already manifested in reality.

Whether reprogramming your own subconscious mind or asking the Creator, keep the images and words positive and in the present tense. To do otherwise is to reprogram or pray against instead of for.

## The Huna System of Prayer

In the Huna philosophy, which is a modern Western interpretation of traditional Hawaiian practices, effective prayer goes from the conscious mind to the subconscious, which energizes that prayer and sends it to the superconscious—or from your middle self to your low self to your high self. This can be done with controlled breathing, affirmation, and visualization all at once. Several of my spiritual teachers—independently of each other—told me how powerful and effective this Huna technique of prayer is.[48]

The man who founded the Huna system and wrote many books on the subject during the twentieth century was Max Freedom Long. Although the traditional Kahuna magician priests of Hawaii during the 1800s would not readily share their inner teachings with the white

---

[47] **Search Phrase: Christine Sheldon—*How to Change Your Frequency to Change your Life.***
[48] **Search Phrases: Huna, Max Freedom Long, healing with Huna.**

invaders, as time passed, a dictionary of their language was developed. The dictionary was thought to include the words used in their mystical practices. Max Long just did his research, working backward from the definitions of words to beliefs and practices. He produced a system for people in the West to use effectively based on what he believed were the ancient Hawaiian beliefs and practices. He passed away in 1971, and Huna has since become a big thing in the New Age movement.

There is no shortage of controversy about Huna, and it is attacked by several academics as being an appropriation of Hawaiian culture, which they claim is often incorrect in its usage of Hawaiian terminology. Although Huna currently has many enthusiastic adherents and proponents, if interested, I suggest reading what was written by Max Freedom Long. Some of his later followers get way out there, so you may want to stick with Long's originals for an effective and simple system of prayer. New and used copies of his books are available on the net.

The Huna system of prayer is often used by people because it is a simple, effective, and basic system that fits popular psychology's breakdown of the three aspects of being. Huna teaches that prayer should start as an image/phrase in the ego/conscious mind/middle self, should be energized by the unconscious/subconscious mind/low self, and then sent up to the superego/superconscious mind/high self, which will powerfully manifest the image into reality.

For healing, one develops the image of perfect health in the middle self; that image is energized by the low self by using controlled breathing or combining the image with the feeling one has when getting ready to run a race and sending that energized image up to the high self.

The traditional Indians, Chinese, and Japanese postulated chakras, energy fields, and meridians. Long centered the low self in the solar plexus, the middle self in the brain, and the high self above the head—all connected by the energy of their energy fields (mana, mana mana, and mana loa). Thus, one imagines the prayer/image going from the head down to be energized in the solar plexus and then sent up to the high self above the head.

Some of the current Huna adherents are very New Age, and at least a few on the net are pretty far out there. I have already mentioned how decades ago, while Huna was still just what Max Long wrote, several of my teachers indicated that his system of prayer was simple, powerful, and effective when done correctly. His original books are still available.

If you practice this system do not think you are practicing the system used by Hawaiian magician-priests three hundred years ago or by today's traditional Kahunas. This is a Western system, based on one man's investigation and interpretation of ancient beliefs which he melded with some modern ones. Even if some of the criticism of his work is academically correct, that doesn't mean his prayer technique is not extremely effective.

Huna continues to be used by so many adherents because it is such a simple system of prayer. The middle self, low self, and high self of Huna match very well modern psychology's conscious, subconscious, and superconscious minds. Because it equates so well with what you already know, it is easy to use.

## Meditation

Some people consider prayer and meditation to be very similar activities. Others would argue the point. I don't care where you come down on this argument. Maybe you are a believer in a higher spiritual power, and you pray every day for others and then for yourself. Maybe you are a nonbeliever. Whether you are a believer in a higher power or not, you can meditate each day. Consider the large body of scientific research; it generally indicates that meditation is very healthy and good for you. However, meditation is a general term covering myriad techniques.[49]

Go to Wikipedia or any respectable and dependable source and get familiar with the field in general; investigate its history, and the scientific research into its many benefits. There is little doubt that done safely and correctly, most forms of meditation reduce stress and anxiety and promote relaxation and a state of well-being. Science has proven meditation can change the brain waves and state of consciousness of the practitioner from everyday normal beta to meditative alpha, and with practice or talent move to deeper delta, and some even into theta, your normal deep sleep state.

---

[49] **Search Phrases: meditation, the benefits of meditation.**

I personally have always been drawn to the moving forms of meditation and those that use sound to affect the body and mind.

## Life-Force Building Meditations

If you examine the history of meditation, you find the practice was highly
developed in the East, but most cultures and religions have developed
some system of meditation.

Certain forms of meditation are really concentration; some are con-
templation. There is a wide variety to choose from. Find a time every day
when you can practice without being disturbed. Whatever meditation
you choose, it should relax your body and foster deep rhythmic breathing.

Some types of meditation are moving forms of meditation and were
developed to enhance health and build internal energy or life force. This
pervasive concept of a life force is known in India as prana, in China,
Korea, and Japan as Chi, Qi, or Ki, in Hawaii as Mana, and fictionally in
*Star Wars* as the Force. (Some sources capitalize all these energy names,
others do not.)

Most forms of yoga build prana and contain an element of meditation. Tai Chi and Qi Gong or Chi Kung build your Chi or Qi and are
health-boosting forms of moving meditation. This concept of using your
body, deep breathing, and mind to increase your life force and ensure its
free flow are central to the philosophies of health in India, China, and
Japan—as well as to the practice of acupuncture and other Eastern and
Western healing arts.

Many forms of Qi Gong are used to fight disease and restore health.
I like the site on YouTube titled "Healing and Cancer—Qi Gong." There
is also what is known as medical Qi Gong. As long as you continue with
the best of modern medicine, diet, and the rest of my program, do all the
Qi Gong or yoga you want.[50]

---

[50] **Search Phrases: Life force, prana, Qi or Chi, Ki, Mana; yoga, Tai Chi, Qi
Gong, Do-in; Medical Qi Gong, on YouTube "Healing and Cancer—Qi Gong."**

## Sound and Vibrations in Meditation and Healing

We talked earlier about the sixties and seventies and the concept of good and bad vibes and raising one's vibes. In the New Age movement, it is often referred to as raising one's frequency. If you find a form of meditation that suits you and you do it correctly, your body should become relaxed, and you should breathe deeply. With regular practice, it should greatly reduce immune-inhibiting stress, fear, and anxiety. Your brain waves should move from beta to alpha and enhance a feeling of well-being. This is raising one's vibes.

For tens of thousands of years, mystics have known that sound can affect the human mind and body. Most people would agree and have experienced how melodies, rhythms, and songs can affect emotions. It would be difficult to find a culture or religion that does not use words, sounds, chanting, singing, percussion, or music to affect the body-mind-spirit. Tibetans use bowls, others in the East use gongs, and cultures everywhere use drums or other percussive sounds ritually and in their spiritual pursuits.[51]

If you search "healing sounds," you will find various examples of healing sounds, including Tibetan bowls and belief in the use of the 528 Hz sounds and the interesting work of Dr. Len Horowitz. There are many good sites concerning the power of sound to heal, and I encourage the reader to explore this field fully.

## Healing Sounds

Sound is central to some healing philosophies. There are New Age healers who use tuning forks to try to heal the body-mind-spirit. There is the work of Dr. Len Horowitz, the belief in the healing properties of certain frequencies, especially 528 hertz, and their relation to the Solfeggio and the Fibonacci numerical sequences and patterns which are found throughout nature. When you Google this, there will be plenty of information and an abundance of debate.

Dr. Len Horowitz is a highly controversial figure with many books

---

[51] **Search Phrases: healing sounds.**

and a website, and he presents a complete and coherent philosophy. Examples of people utilizing his work with the 528 Hz sounds and the Solfeggio and Fibonacci sequences can be found in abundance on YouTube. Do your own research. Sample the various sites featuring this healing music. If you are getting the best modern medical help, following the best diet, and working the rest of the eight-part plan, if it is free and you believe in it, use it. I certainly don't know how listening to it could hurt anything, and some of Horowitz's followers think it is powerfully healing and can mend damaged DNA.[52]

On YouTube, you can find sites that play this healing music for hours. There are eight-hour versions for you to sleep and heal with. Some of the music, sounds, and sequences are to work on certain specific problems. Find the music that matches what you want to work on. It can't hurt, and it might help. The average doctor won't get it—so don't even bring it up with your doctor. If it feels healing to you, and you are drawn to it, then listen and heal.

## The Science of Cymatics

To see the proof of how sound affects matter, check out the science of Cymatics on YouTube. If you have any doubt that sound can affect matter, you can perform an experiment I used in elementary school and high school. It was incorrectly called an ediphone. An ediphone was one of Thomas Edison's first telephones. The device I used for my science projects looked something like the speaking apparatus of Edison's phone. I got a large metal coffee can, attached a funnel to a metal tube, and stuck it into the side of the can at an upward angle. I stretched a cut-up balloon over the top of the can and secured it with a rubber band. I sprinkled sand on top, sang different notes into the funnel, and watched the sand forming consistent patterns. This primitive form of Cymatics got me two As and instilled in me the strong belief that sound could affect matter.

Today's New Age movement points out how the average adult is 55–60 percent water, and water is easily and visibly affected by sound. Some

---

[52] **Search Phrases: Dr. Len Horowitz, 528 hertz, and the Solfeggio and Fibonacci sequences.**

of the most visually dramatic Cymatic experiments are done with sound and water. If you have the least bit of an open mind, watch the Cymatics videos on YouTube. If it is scientifically proven that sound can physically affect water, which it has—and your body is 60 percent water, which it is—then sound can hurt or heal your body. Our military uses sound as a weapon. If sound can be used to hurt, it can also be used to help.[53]

## The Power of Words and Intention

You really must put in some hours on the internet. There are interesting science-based articles and videos on YouTube; there is slightly far-out stuff and some highly questionable stuff. Use your powers of discernment and find what suits you.

Those with New Age leanings are probably already familiar with the work of Dr. Masaru Emoto and his photos of water crystals showing the power of words/vibrations used with intention. Ugly words produce ugly ice crystals; healing and uplifting words and phrases create beautiful ice crystals.

Although his work is controversial and not repeated yet in double-blind studies, his photos of ice crystals affected by words used with intention are so captivating they are now known around the world. I was lent his book by a friend, and it truly has some amazing photographs. Look him up on Google and decide for yourself.

Since you are mostly water molecules, and the vibrations of words—either written or spoken with intention—seem to have a powerful effect on water molecules, then it could easily be extrapolated that words with intention can have a powerful effect on you and your environment. Words written or spoken with intention may have very real healing power—like in your affirmations.[54]

After reading Dr. Emoto's book, I was convinced it couldn't hurt and could very possibly help, so I used his techniques. His book indicated that some of the most powerful human vibrations are those of joyful gratitude. On a piece of paper, with strong intention, I wrote: "Thank God for

---

[53] **Search Phrases: science of Cymatics, sound as a weapon.**
[54] **Search Phrases: Dr. Masaru Emoto, books by Masaru Emoto.**

becoming perfectly healthy, well, and whole." I put it on my bedside table under my nighttime water. It is still there.

## My Shotgun Approach to Self-Healing

According to the ideas of the late Dr. Emoto, when I set my water on top of that paper, the water was absorbing the vibrations, the idea, and the intention of joyful thanks for perfect health. Now as mystical and as hard as that may be to prove scientifically, can science prove that it had no beneficial effect?

I want you to feel free to follow your personal interests as long as you continue to

- use the best of modern medicine,
- follow the best diet, and
- work the rest my eight-part program.
- If it doesn't hurt anyone or anything—even if science and medicine say it is absolutely nothing but the placebo effect, if it is free or you can easily afford it, and if it is something *you believe will help you*, it very well may help.

When facing this disease, I believe in the shotgun approach. The metaphor is that the disease is a rabid animal that needs to be put down, and you will kill that rabid animal with your self-healing shotgun. You load your self-healing shotgun shells with the buckshot pellets of everything you think will or might possibly work and fire it at the disease. The buckshot pellets in your self-healing shotgun shells include modern medicine, the best diet, visualization, the rest of my eight-part plan, and anything else (harmless) you believe in. You fire your buckshot at the target. All the buckshot doesn't have to hit the target—as long as some of the pellets kill the disease.

## Kotodama

Dr. Emoto believed he showed what intention and words can do; the Cymatics videos show what sound can do. Some of the 528 Hz YouTube video/music tracks are extremely pleasing to play in the background. Make sound your ally, learn to chant in the shower, make it a pleasing and joyful sound, and use sound however you can in your self-healing program.

You may want to go to Wikipedia and look up *kototama* or *kotodama*. This is an important concept in Japanese mysticism. You will find this concept in the martial art aikido and in the many works of Michio Kushi. They believe that words and sounds affect matter and that words used ritually can affect the environment. There is a rough analogy here to some of the beliefs of the Kabbalah.

This concept that words and sounds can affect the environment and the body-mind-spirit can be found all over the world. Often there will be a symbolic meaning ascribed to the letters of the alphabet and to certain numbers in such philosophies. Hebrew and Sanskrit and other ancient languages follow this model. In many such ancient cultures, the name of God describes the process of creation. God speaks the creative word, and the world comes into being.[55]

Other than the concept that sounds, words, and words written or spoken with strong intentions can affect your healing, the study of sacred languages, sacred letters, and sacred numbers is not all that relevant to our self-healing program unless they are part of your heritage or otherwise of interest to you. If you search for these subjects on the net, you will find some interesting, some questionable, and some ridiculous stuff.

## Using Sound in Meditation and for Healing

It is interesting to go from religion to religion, culture to culture, including vastly distant lands, and find similar sounds used in religion, meditation, and healing. If you are Christian, you often say amen, elsewhere in the Middle East, it is amin, like the Indian aum or om, similar to the

---

[55] **Search Phrases: the healing power of words, kotodama.**

Egyptian "Amoun Ra." If you Google this, you will find many interesting articles. I personally have found similarities in the Buddhist use of chanting "hum" (who-uuu-ummm) and the Native American "Shu(uuu)" in the first part of a cleansing chant. Both are used as healing sounds that sweep away negative energy and clear the way for healing.

When we talked about raising one's vibes, I mentioned singing in the bathtub or shower where the tile and close walls help intensify the sound effects. It does the same thing very effectively with chanting. In some religions they chant a mantra, a sound, word, or phrase over and over. This can be a name of God, sounded repeatedly. In some forms of meditation, a healing word or uplifting sound such as *aum*, *om*, or *hum* is repeated over and over. Sometimes a phrase is repeated over and over.

There are complete systems of yoga that are mantra yoga. Everywhere around the world, you can find the use of sound to raise and heal the human body-mind-spirit. I believe emphatically that meaningfully chanting or singing (whatever is comfortable to you) while bathing each day helps heal the body-mind-spirit.

With the science of Cymatics, you can visibly see how easily sound can affect water. Think of your body as a 60 percent water tuning fork and use singing or chanting. Around the world, sounds and phrases have been used for healing for hundreds or thousands of years.

## Chanting Aum or Amen

Readers who are not New Age might have never chanted and might not know where to start. Wikipedia has a section that teaches you how to do things, and they have a section on how to chant the aum sound. It was not exactly how I learned, but I tried their technique and thought it was excellent. If your religion keeps you within narrow constraints, you must do what feels comfortable and follow your traditions and beliefs. However, most religions have pleasing and healing songs, chants, mantras, prayers, or chanting the name of God which could be repeated while bathing or showering. If you are chanting a powerful traditional healing sound while bathing, the science of Cymatics proves you are having some measurable effect on the water in your tub and on the 60 percent of your body that is water.[56]

Think about how your body being 60 percent water helps make you a giant tuning fork. By chanting aum, amen, aum-om-hum, om mani padme om, the name of your God, or whatever you are drawn to or your tradition dictates, you are creating and tuning in to a healing sound. This is meditation, self-healing, and vibe raising all at the same time. For thousands of years, mystics have believed that very real physical healing can be brought about through the use of sound and words.[57]

There is a form of Buddhism from Japan that has as a central core the teaching of chanting Nam-myoho-renge-kyo to burn off negative karma. My understanding of the concept is that when the bad karma is burned off, the person returns to a state of health.

## Load Up with Sound

You can adopt my shotgun approach and load the use of sound into your self-healing shotgun shells, along with the best modern medical care, the best diet, visualization, affirmation, exercising, and raising your vibes. One of the easiest and most effective ways of raising your vibes may be using sound while bathing.

Chanting is a form of healing meditation. For those readers who are open-minded and unconstrained by conservative or fundamentalists beliefs, you can chant aum or other mantras and affect the 60 percent of your body which is water (and the rest of your body) raising those vibes. Many religions will practice the repetition of a mystical name of God. There are simple one-sound or one-word chants and more complex healing mantras. Among them are some simple chants—aum, om, hum and other single-sentence mantras from Japan and Tibet. You can find many options on the internet. *Om mani padme hum* is an example.

Some chants are a nonreligious use of sound, while some religions may claim ownership and have religious beliefs built around certain mantras or names for God. Some in India may be emphatic that a certain

[56] **Search Phrase: chanting the name of God.**
[57] **Search Phrase on YouTube: How to chant aum, Healing Chants, Nam-myoho-renge-kyo.**

sound is the creative word of God. Many religions have this idea. The variety can be vast, but nobody owns a healing sound or chant. Trust your intuition, find what appeals to you, learn how to chant, and immediately raise the vibes of the 60 percent of your being that is water, which raises the vibes of your whole body. I implore you to do everything you can to supercharge your immune system and actualize all your inner self-healing mechanisms.

Learn to use the healing names, chants, or sounds you find on the internet, in a yoga class, or from whatever source is available to you as part of your self-healing regime. Learn to chant, loudly, fully, and without inhibition in the shower or tub.[58]

If you are a one-way Christian or an adherent of some other fundamentalist outlook, you can chant the appropriate name of God or just sing the songs that inspire you and raise your vibes. You might follow that by singing and repeating amen, amin, or your version of that closing. By emphasizing the first syllable, you are using sound to raise your vibes.

Your personal religious beliefs are yours, and I've tried to write for all people, religious or not. Chanting the name(s) of God can be a very meaningful and powerful experience for some. Even if you are just using a pleasing sound, if this weakens the enemies of your immune system—stress and anxiety—thereby strengthening your immune system, you are raising your vibes and participating in self-healing. You are combining your meditation, bathing, and the beneficent use of sound.

## Keep Combining Techniques

Bathing every day is a healthy and uplifting habit when fighting an illness. The mystics believe that bathing cleans more than just your body. Every day, you can sing uplifting spiritual songs or chant while in the tub or shower as a self-healing meditation. Defeating disease—becoming free and clear and healthy—can be a full-time job, so combining healing activities is important. Every day, bathe or shower and chant, sing, or lift a joyful voice unto the Lord. Whatever you feel comfortable doing, raise your vibes every chance you get.

---

[58] **Search Phrases: How to chant aum, Om, mani padme hum.**

We cannot underestimate the power of words and sounds. In many spiritual traditions, the Creator speaks the creative word and gives rise to the universe. In the Bible, we are taught that in the beginning was the Word, the Word was with God, and the Word was God. God spoke the creative Word of God and gave rise to the universe. My limited understanding of traditional Hebrew belief would be that this was the tetragrammaton, which is the creative Word of God.

In India, they are pretty sure that creative word sounded like aum. The aum sound is now highly recommended all around the world. If you aren't comfortable chanting aum, look up the meaning of amen. If you are Christian and uncomfortable with aum, state one of your self-healing affirmations and then repeatedly sing or chant amen. You might say, "I am now, and I am become perfectly health, well, and whole," and then chant amen ten times.

Whatever faith or philosophy you follow, find an appropriate name, healing sound, or healing song and sing or chant it when you bathe. Done correctly, this is a mantra meditation and a combined self-healing/vibe-raising session.

# CHAPTER 9 |||||

## Exercising—Western and Eastern

This book is designed to be utilized as quickly after diagnosis as possible while the patient is in the beginning stages of the struggle. Some of what I am proposing is not applicable to people who through no fault of their own show up late for the dance. Since this is a disease with many cases of spontaneous remission at almost every stage of the disease, I don't believe in ever giving up all hope.

How one lives or leaves this life is every individual's choice and decision. Each person has the right to decide for herself or himself. For those who have fought this battle for some time, if conventional modern medicine's repeated rounds of radiation and chemo have weakened and poisoned the patient's body—and more rounds are predicted to buy very limited time—they should do what they think is best. Don't let people guilt-trip you into spending the last few weeks of your life being poisoned in the hospital if you don't want to—spend those last few weeks as you choose.

Don't misunderstand when I call radiation and chemo poison. Although these treatments are becoming much more targeted, in the simplest and most general terms, the whole theory of both treatments is that mutant cells are weaker than normal healthy cells, so the radiation or chemo kills the mutant cells first. This is somewhat similar to the Warburg effect, which shows that mutant cells live only on sugar and starve to death on ketones. Mutant cells are different than normal cells; they are weaker than normal cells, use sugar quicker, and often replicate rapidly. That is why I implore the patient to move quickly in all facets of the healing process.

## Moving toward Life or Embracing Death

Whenever I counsel someone fighting a serious illness or injury, I try to make it simple. I tell them there are always and only two directions you can choose in life. You can move toward health and well-being or you can move toward unhealth and death. If you are fighting this disease, you can get the best medical treatment available, deeply breathe clean air, drink pure water, eat clean healthy food, take the right vitamins and supplements, use visualization and affirmation, pray, meditate, chant in the bathtub, raise your vibes, and exercise. This is moving toward life. Or you can ignore all medical and well-meaning advice, drink, smoke, get no exercise, sit around, watch TV, and then lay there and die. That is moving toward death. Either way, this movement can only originate from within the patient.

My brother battled leukemia for many years. Being part Indian and appreciating Native American culture, he had always embraced a saying made famous during the Indian versus European invader wars: "Hokahey, today is a good day to die." I disagreed strongly, telling him no day was a good day to die and that he needed to fight in every way possible. He finally embraced that idea a few weeks before he passed, but it was way too late.

At the time of his final struggle, and in the years immediately following his passing, better medications became available. My sister-in-law and I have wondered if he had done all the good things in the paragraph above and none of the bad things, would it have bought him enough time to be there when the better meds became available? If he had fought differently, might he still be alive today?

I have a cousin who was fighting a different manifestation of cancer around the same time I was. I can't help but wonder if he had this book and had worked it diligently from the day he was diagnosed, would he still be alive?

I can't let these questions haunt me. All I can do is get this book to diagnosed readers as soon as possible, while they can still exercise and aggressively implement the rest of my program.


## Concerning Life and Death

When dealing with questions surrounding life and death, one thought that provided me some relief was remembering something Grandmother Eve told me once when I asked her the perennial spiritual questions of how much is predetermined in our lives and how much is free will. She was of the opinion that the day we were born, the day we pass away, and maybe the day we are married were determined before we came into manifestation. She thought pretty much everything else was free will. Remembering this has brought me some solace concerning the passing of my cousin, my brother, and my parents.

When it comes to moving toward life or death, we must accept the fact that not everyone is meant to, or designed to, reach ninety or one hundred. Some people have an intuitive knowing that their time to pass has come. There is no complete medical cure for this disease in the immediate future. Without vast scientific and medical improvements, I don't expect 100 percent of the people who read and work this book to get well. In nature, people live and die. For some people, it is simply their time—and this disease is the mechanism that takes them.

If you are an elderly person who is satisfied and at peace with your life, and you have a deep intuitive knowledge that your time is up, then go gracefully in the manner that you choose. If those are not your circumstances, fight with everything you have. If you have children who need you, if your affairs are not in order, or if you have unfinished business here on earth, fight with everything you have.


## Exercising and Support Groups

Both Western and Eastern forms of exercise represent moving toward life. If you are healthy enough, do calisthenics and other cardiovascular exercises, and work out with weights; use light or very light dumbbells if nothing else. Get your circulation going, get your lungs working, and drink purified water. If you go online, you will find the many ways exercise can boost your immune system—as long as it is moderate, not extreme, and you get plenty of rest and adequate nutrition.

This would be a good time to go online and put into your search engine the following:

- "How much exercise should a cancer patient get each week?"
- "cancer and activity"
- "cancer and exercise"

Myriad articles will show up from respectable sources, listing as many as fourteen advantages to exercising while fighting this disease. There are factors that must be considered as you develop your exercise program, including the type and stage of the disease, the treatments you are undergoing, and your previous level of fitness, strength, and activity. If you go through the various articles, they will give you an idea of what to do. Read and follow the guidelines and precautions.[59]

Most of these articles will repeat the idea that they want you to be as active as possible and continue your previous level of activity. You should continue or begin exercising at an intelligent moderate level daily, with possible strength (weight or resistance) training twice weekly or every other day. When you put into your search engine "exercise programs for cancer patients," there will be books and programs with plenty of diagrams for those with little exercise experience.

You will read recommendations that advise you to return to your normal activity level immediately after diagnosis. Your level of activity and exercise after diagnosis must be relative to that before diagnosis. If you have been exercising, read, study, and keep it up. If you have been sedentary, that may be one reason you got the disease—and you need to change your lifestyle. This should be done gradually and with moderation. If you've sat in your lounge chair for the last twenty years watching TV, drinking, and smoking, do not immediately attempt training to run a marathon. Gradually build your activity level, strength, and endurance.

Exercising while undergoing treatment will vastly improve your

---

[59] **Search Phrases: How much exercise should a cancer patient get each week, Cancer and activity, Cancer and exercise.**

quality of life. Once you are free and clear, exercise is as important as before to ensure your quality of life and that you remain free and clear. Exercise is considered extremely important to prevent any disease recurrence. The September 2015 magazine from DeKalb Medical's *Pushing Beyond* has an article titled "Exercise and Your Options." It states that the American Cancer Society and the CDC have recommended that cancer survivors get 150 minutes of low-intensity or 75 minutes of vigorous activity a week plus two strength-training sessions.

This level of exercise helps patients to deal with the postsurgical changes in their bodies and some of the side effects of treatment like neuropathy, lymphedema (limb swelling), joint pain, and fatigue. This workout schedule leads to improvements in strength, pain control, energy levels, and mental outlook. One of the most important points was that the participants came to see their exercise classes as a support group that works out together. While recovering from my second and more major surgery, I worked out daily in bed with five-pound dumbbells. I just did curls and presses, but it made me feel better during the extremely gross and uncomfortable postsurgical recovery months. I would constantly remind myself of the joy of being free and clear and that all the discomfort would pass in six to ten weeks.

I had been told by several doctors that because I had used the suprapubic catheter for decades, there were multiple colonies of infections in my bladder that would never go away. Although these colonies of infections were under control by my immune system (unless I became stressed or run down), that situation and some squamous cells in the bladder wall meant it was best if it went. At that point in time, for my peace of mind, I agreed. They removed my bladder and replaced it with an ileal conduit.

The joy of being free and clear made up for all the inconveniences and aesthetic negatives that came with the ileal conduit. Before I had a suprapubic catheter, and now I had an urostomy. It was a change, but not that big a change, and I was alive, free, and clear. If I had an integrative oncologist from the very beginning and more dietary guidance, with what I know now, I might have chosen to see if my diet could have eliminated all the mutant cells once the tumor was eliminated and found to be benign. Even if I had done that, the continued use of the suprapubic catheter would have been a constant source of concern. The peace of mind I got once they cut it all out, and my body was free and clear, was profound.

## The Necessity for Support

One of the first things I do when I counsel the ill or injured is look for their support group. If I go into a hospital room filled with friends and family who are trying to be upbeat and supportive, I don't worry. However, not everyone lives near their friends and family. You may have taken a job far away from your family and friends and then come down with the disease. If you are fighting for your life and are not surrounded by family and friends, you need to go to one or more support groups regularly. Human beings are very social animals. By going to support groups, you will come to understand you are not the only person going through such an extreme challenge on both an emotional and mental level.

Even if you have a good family/friend support network, you may want to go to a support group just to be around others going through something similar to your struggle. Each person is unique, but you may learn much from others who have gone through it and become survivors—and you may have much to teach others. Under no circumstances should anyone try to fight this disease by themselves.[60]

As mentioned above, if you can find an exercise class for people fighting this disease and for survivors, it can become a support group as well as an exercise class.

## Defeating Depression with Exercise and Positive Activity

Some people teach that the body repairs and heals itself best while sleeping. When fighting an illness, adequate rest and getting enough sleep is extremely important.

Of course, there is a big difference between getting adequate sleep and being depressed and staying in bed all day. All the self-healing techniques in this book are aimed at improving health, well-being, and boosting the immune system. It is hard for me to believe that if one begins soon

---

[60] **Search Phrase: the importance of cancer support groups.**

enough after diagnosis and applies all these techniques, they will be the kind of person who stays in bed all day, depressed.

For one thing, the motivated self-healers will be way too busy getting fresh, clean organic food, taking vitamins and supplements, weighing, measuring, and preparing their food, doing Western and Eastern forms of exercise, praying, meditating, using visualization and affirmation, bathing, singing or chanting, and raising their vibes to stay in bed and be depressed. I believe the two are exclusive of each other. Only one of those two behavior models will help you to go to sleep, tired, each night, knowing you have done your part and that you deserve to get well.

## Develop Your Own Personal Exercise Program

Every person battling this disease is unique, and there is no one-size-fits all exercise program available on the internet. Talk to your doctor. Maybe all you can do is go for a walk each day. Maybe all you can do is sit in a chair and exercise with one-pound dumbbells. At most stages of this struggle, there are some exercises you can do.

This disease has myriad manifestations, but all doctors would agree the earlier the diagnosis and beginning of treatment the better. This disease definitely has a tipping point at which it becomes so progressed it is difficult to recover from despite whatever therapy is employed.

This program is designed to be utilized with an early diagnosis; for those who find this program later than desired, the exercise options may be limited, but deep breathing is almost always good for one and helps raise the oxygen level in the blood. Always talk to your doctor and other health care professionals concerning your exercise program and what is appropriate for your individual situation. Seek second and third opinions if necessary. You may want to join an exercise class at a regular gym or go to one specifically for patients with this disease. When you search "exercise programs + fighting cancer," there will be many options. Although I personally had a bad experience at MD Anderson, they have an excellent reputation and a good exercise guide on the net.[61]

---

[61] **Search Phrase: exercise programs + fighting cancer.**

## Monitor Yourself Honestly

Wherever you are in the fight—for health, for your life—you must monitor yourself honestly. Don't push yourself too hard, but don't be lazy. How you sleep at night and how you feel the next day should be your feedback mechanisms when it comes to exercise.

Anyone who hasn't been exercising and then begins might have some aches and pains. This is normal. What you choose to do in the way of your exercise program can also be affected by personal preferences and affordability. You may already be doing a sport, be in an exercise program, or be a member of a gym. If not, you may want to join one, get a personal trainer, download a program from the web, or get a book at the library. There is no shortage of information or options when it comes to exercise.

I recently spoke to a woman who had played tennis at a high amateur level the whole time she fought the disease. She told me it helped her make it through. She played with a scarf when she had no hair. She also emphasized how important group support was in the process.

## Western and Eastern Exercise

If you have gone online and put in the suggested phrases, you've seen the abundance of Western cardiovascular and weight-training exercise programs. Your library will also have plenty of books on the subject. If you've been living a sedentary lifestyle and want to begin an exercise program, don't overdo it. Start with a few exercises and add in a few more every week as you get in better shape. Start with short walks and make them longer until it's at least a half-hour walk each day. Most people have some experience with Western-style exercise programs. Fewer will have experience with an Eastern form.

There is no shortage of information and videos on YouTube concerning the following:

- yoga
- yoga for fighting cancer
- Qi Gong for fighting cancer

- medical Qi Gong
- Tai Chi

There is some but much less information available on Do-in, which is a shiatsu, self-massage, meridian stretching, and deep-breathing exercise system. Yoga practice has gone mainstream in the United States; the others are more prevalent in cities and areas with large Asian populations.[62]

Any of these life force-building exercise systems can help you. You can sample various YouTube videos and find what you like. You can try more than one of these systems and combine exercises you like into a personal workout. Some of these exercises can be relatively short—see various examples of Dragon-Tiger medical Qi Gong—or they can be long and extended workouts. There are many excellent videos on YouTube—or you can buy DVDs. I like the "healing and cancer—Qi Gong" exercise video on YouTube.[63]

The only caution I would give here is to listen to informed advice and listen to your own intuition. You want the mutant cells to stay where they are and be destroyed by your immune system. Everything I am guiding you to do has the simple purpose of holding the bad cells in place, and these diet, medical treatments, and self-healing activities empower your immune system to kill all the aberrant cells, allowing your body to replace them with normal healthy cells. If any exercise, yoga form, Qi Gong movement, or massage makes you feel like it is working against keeping the mutant cells in place, don't do it!

It is your body and your mind; trust your intuition and your feelings.

## Use Common Sense and Intuition

In my own case, the bad cells were only in my bladder. All testing throughout the process indicated they were only in my bladder. There were certain Qi Gong moves I absolutely refused to do as I battled the disease. I would not breathe and visualize the movement of energy through my challenged bladder to the healthy parts of my body. Agnostics or atheists

---

[62] **Search Phrases: Qi Gong + healing cancer, Dragon and Tiger Medical Qi Gong, yoga + healing cancer, Medical Qi Gong.**
[63] **Search Phrase: healing and cancer—Qi Gong.**

may laugh at this notion, but if it made me uncomfortable, why would I do it?

If you feel like any massage technique, yoga position, Tai Chi form, Qi Gong exercise, or anything at all is working against keeping the mutant cells in place and inactive, don't do it! Stop it immediately—no matter what the situation is. It is your body; embarrassment is nothing compared to health and peace of mind. Always follow your intuition in every part of this process.

## Building Healthy Habits

When it comes to exercise, it is a question of finding what is appropriate for your individual situation, finding what you like to do so you'll do it, having the self-discipline to begin doing it, and building up the habit of doing it.

I heard about a study that indicated as much as 80 percent of human behavior was habitual and done without conscious thought or volition. I was shocked, but it also awakened me to the possibility of the power of good habits. Although it isn't necessarily easy to change our old habits, we can establish new patterns in a short period of time. If you have been a person with many unhealthy habits, that may help explain why you are fighting this disease and need this book. Once you have been diagnosed, it may be late, but it's not too late to stop unhealthy habits and replace them with healthy habits.

## Fighting the Disease while Raising Kids and/or Working

You may be working and/or raising kids while you are going through this struggle. Nobody in their right mind thinks it is easy for you. If you are going through the stress of disease with work and/or kids, try to remember what is good for the immune system and what inhibits it. In general, exercise with adequate rest and sleep, good nutrition, and adequate oxygen in the blood are good for you and strengthen the immune system. Insufficient rest, bad nutrition, low oxygen levels, stress, and anxiety are bad for you and inhibit the immune system. Even if you have had bad habits in the past, you now have the knowledge, the tools, and the impetus to correct your bad habits and replace them with healthy habits.

My self-healing system is a full-time job in and of itself. When you add in a job, raising children, or both, you have a lot—maybe too much—on your plate. Wherever you go for modern medical treatment, they should be able to fix you up with a support group to attend. An oncology social worker may be able to help you with the child-raising issues. Take advantage of all the help offered to you. Don't ever be too proud to take advantage of whatever help is available. Such help may be available but not be offered, and you may have to ask for it.[64]

---

[64] **Search Phrase: fighting cancer + raising children, fighting caner + while working, oncology social workers.**

# CHAPTER 10

# Radical Remission

## Spontaneous or Radical Remission

When I was diagnosed, I was aware that cases of spontaneous remission had been documented at all stages of this disease so I did not research the subject. I arrogantly assumed that I knew about it, accepted it as real for whatever unknown percentage of patients, and researched what I had no knowledge of—like the twelve-gram disease-starvation diet, vitamins and supplements to fight bladder mutations, etc. Once I had gone through my treatment and been free and clear for a few years, I decided to write the book I wish I had gotten my hands on the day I was diagnosed. I was well into writing this book and had pretty much told my story when I googled "spontaneous remission + cancer" for the first time. I was absolutely amazed. I felt at that moment what I'd only experienced once before in my life.

I wrote *Crime and the Disabled* to cover the field of personal safety, crime prevention, and self-defense for the disabled and an accompanying instructional manual (*The We Defend System Manual*). They are both available from Lulu.com and from my website for disabled self-defense *thewedefendsystem.org* for anyone interested. My Sifu, or karate father, Master Robert Quinn, and I worked on developing our techniques for a decade. Then I saw a *National Geographic* special on TV that was scientifically testing the techniques of self-defense as taught by some of the foremost experts in the field—a male policeman of thirty years, a female policewoman of twenty years who specialized in rape prevention, and a retired Navy SEAL. What they taught concerning able-bodied self-defense was a complete confirmation of everything Master Quinn and I taught. To know that the concepts and principles you worked for a decade to develop are verified by the most respected experts in the field is a huge relief, a big confidence builder, and a deep internal yes!

That same feeling of verification was exactly what I experienced after writing about 70 percent of this book and then discovering the work of Dr. Kelly Turner, PhD. She is the leading researcher in the field of spontaneous remission and has correctly renamed it *radical remission*. She will be the first to admit that spontaneous remissions occur in all types and phases of this disease; but far more of her cases are remissions that occur over extended periods of time.

Dr. Turner examined more than a thousand documented serious cases where patients should be dead or had been given weeks, months, or years to live. Those she studied were 80 percent free and clear, and the rest still had the disease in their body, but in a very reduced, stable, and manageable form. Although there are rare cases of people who prayed, went to a religious healing service, or to a spiritual healer and were healed overnight, most of the radical remissions she studied occurred over weeks, months, or years.[65]

## The Nine Principles of Radical Remission

In the thousand cases of radical remission—of people literally brought back from the edge of death against all odds—she grouped them into three types and discovered nine common principles used by these people to obtain a radical remission. Radical remissions happened for people in three groups:

- people who never used modern medicine and used only alternative treatments
- people who used modern medicine and went alternative when it didn't work
- people who combined modern medicine with alternative therapies

---

[65] **Search Phrase: Dr. Kelly Turner + radical remission.**

She found nine principles in the thousand cases of radical remission:

- changing of one's diet
- taking control over one's health
- following one's intuition
- using herbs and supplements
- releasing suppressed emotions
- increasing positive emotions
- seeking social support
- deepening of spiritual life
- having a strong reason for living

Trust Your Intuition

I agree wholeheartedly with the results of her study. They reify what I have been teaching with the one exception that I have been remiss in not mentioning earlier and will cover in the next section. One point she covers that I have mentioned several times, but probably not enough, is the importance of trusting and following one's intuition in every step of the treatment/self-healing process. This is extremely important. Trust your intuition—it can save your life.

The interested reader can easily acquire Dr. Turner's *Radical Remission: Surviving Cancer against All Odds* online and can also take her course on the net (www.radicalremission.com). She is easy to find on YouTube. Although my book was mostly written before I discovered her work—and I haven't yet read her book or taken her course—I blindly endorse her work based on her nine principles. I feel like her book and course and my eight-part plan would work well together in self-healing harmony.[66]

When teaching self-defense as a martial artist, I always teach my students to follow their intuition because it can help them to avoid trouble and save their lives. Science may not have found a way to verify intuition but ask any combat veteran or police officer whether intuition can save your life.

---

[66] **Search Phrases: Dr. Kelly A. Turner's *Radical Remission: Surviving Cancer against All Odds* and her online course www.radicalremission.com.**

In the same way soldiers or police officers learn to trust their intuition, so must you. Listen to that little voice, that inner feeling. If your gut tells you no or yes about something in your treatment plan, listen to it.

## Unblock Any Blockages

I wrote this book in a flow of consciousness based on my life experiences. The "releasing of suppressed emotions" is the one idea I was remiss in not mentioning and am thankful to Dr. Turner for pointing it out. If you have emotional/psychological issues in your personal history that you have not dealt with, things that are suppressed or blocked, which inhibit the full function of your psyche, you must deal with them through introspection, self-reflection, group therapy, or individual counseling with a qualified professional.

If you are twisted and torn up inside, it is much more difficult to mobilize your internal self-healing mechanisms. Although science cannot measure the force of the human psyche, very few doctors doubt its focused and directed power.

Issues that affect you deeply, which you have buried and haven't worked through, tie up or block some or much of the energy of your psyche. Your psyche should be 100 percent focused and directed on self-healing, on a powerful all-conquering immune system, and on becoming free and clear. If you have buried issues, losses, sadness, fear, conflicts, or trauma you must face those issues and get healed.

Many of us have things to work through. Many of us have sublimated tragic or challenging events in childhood, adolescence, or even adulthood. The loss of a loved one, divorce or a bitter breakup, economic problems and the accompanying sense of failure, being abused as a child or as an adult—there are so many things that can be too difficult to deal with at that moment. Instead, we push them down as a defense mechanism so that we can continue to function. Most people have had to do this at one time or another in their lives. Ideally when time has passed—and you are strong enough to deal with the problem—you let it surface. Through introspection and reflection, you can come to terms with it and move on. Whatever energy was blocked is now free.

Unfortunately, not everybody works through everything they

sublimate. Many people need counseling. There should never be any shame or stigma in going for psychological help. You should have access through your oncologists to disease-related group therapy. This can be extremely helpful. However, you may have personal issues that require counseling from a psychologist or psychiatrist or need specific issue-related group therapy. You may want to begin with Dr. Turner's online course. She has exercises to help patients work through blockages at home. If you have sublimated issues, blockages in your psyche, you need to work on them so that all your internal self-healing mechanisms can work at full strength.

## Dealing with the Fear

In an attempt to keep this book as short, as to the point, and as positive as possible, I have not dwelled much on the negative aspects that accompany the diagnosis. There are so many negatives you must contend with: fear of death, fear of the ravages the disease can bring, fear or apprehension concerning tests, fear of everything bad that goes with chemo, radiation, or invasive surgeries, and long postsurgical recoveries. You must fight to not let it overwhelm you and lead you into immune-suppressing depression.

Most importantly—you must deal honestly with the fear that comes along with this disease. I tell everyone how fear comes along on a free ride from that first moment of diagnosis. You don't have to pay your doctor a penny for the nagging fear; it comes absolutely free from that first instant.

You cannot let this fear become a mental prison. You must face the fact that anyone would have such fear, that it is perfectly normal, and move on with your duty to yourself to fight the disease and become healthier. At the same time, you cannot tell yourself you have no fear. Of course you do. Anyone in your situation would.

I've heard many times from combat veterans that courage is not an absence of fear; it is accepting that you feel the fear but doing your duty anyway. Your duty here is to yourself: to do what you can to help your immune system and work to become free and clear.

There is an inverse relation between the amount of debilitating fear you feel and how hard you work for self-healing.

- research and locate a good doctor
- develop a solid treatment plan that *you* oversee and that you completely agree with
- change your diet
- take vitamins and supplements
- use visualization and affirmation
- exercise
- begin bathing, chanting, meditating, and raising vibes
- begin doing the complete breath several times a day

By working the plan you can face that fear head-on and say, "I'm doing my part!" Give fear the metaphorical finger and tell it to be gone.

## The Calling

The need for introspection, the need for internal honesty to face the fear involved, and dredging up the courage to fight a serious disease or injury is a process that is often referred to as "the calling" in shamanic cultures. This calling may be for you to live a better, more balanced, more spiritual life. It may go way past that and be a calling for the patient to become a shaman or become a healer. That was how it was for Grandmother Eve Eaton and for me. In conventional Judeo-Christian thought, it is a calling to return to a more righteous and spiritual life.

I agree with Dr. Turner that physical self-healing is most effective without any psychological or emotional blockages. If you have sublimated or are unsuccessfully fighting memories that you mentally buried in the past and refused to deal with—or if you feel an overwhelming fear or apprehension concerning your illness—now would be the time to face these things. If you deal with them honestly and put them to rest, the subconscious can be working 100 percent for self-healing. Part of the calling is the need to deal with the past and the present honestly and courageously.

If dealing with your apprehension or fear concerning the disease or any sublimated issues from your past requires group therapy or individual counseling, then do it. There should never be any shame or embarrassment in going for psychological help. You have a body, a mind, and a spiritual aspect. Each can need healing.

Thank goodness this is something that has changed for the better in our society. We now admire people who recognize they have issues and seek help. Wherever you are fighting this disease, there should be support groups available. Take advantage of them.

This really is the mandatory time for you to deal with any past issues or new issues with fear. Give yourself the best chance for body-mind-spirit healing by having the conscious and subconscious mind working 100 percent on boosting that immune system and enabling all of your self-healing mechanisms to work at full strength.

It is important to study and incorporate Dr. Turner's nine principles of radical remission into your approach; to some extent, we have covered them all. The one thing I might add to Dr. Turner's list would be a strong reason *or desire* to live.


Your New Belief Systems

Dr. Turner also talks about how good meditation is for the body and how five immune-enhancing chemicals are produced by the body while meditating.

Just like the Seyfried and D'Agostino YouTube videos, you absolutely must watch "the Three Principles of Radical Remission with Dr. Kelly Turner" interview by Kris Carr. There are other longer YouTube videos with Dr. Turner as well. The interviewer is Kris Carr of *Crazy, Sexy Cancer* fame and many of you will be interested in her story, her documentary, and her many instructional YouTube videos.[67]

Watch these videos regularly or listen to them in the background while doing household chores to reinforce your new belief system and foster your belief and faith in all you are doing. When a doctor you respect looks you in the eyes and tells you that if you could starve cancer to death, surely they would have told him that in med school, you can look at him confidently and smile. Don't argue with him. Just have the confidence of a Nobel Prize, straight logic, and all the anecdotal evidence of people

---

[67] **Search Phrase on YouTube: "The Three Principles of Radical Remission with Dr. Kelly Turner" interview by Kris Carr.**

who have gotten well—and then *you* prove *him* wrong. Once you are well, explain all you did to become healthy.

What you are doing is backed up by science and common sense, but I believe very strongly in the need to positively reinforce new ideas. This is all unknown or new to many doctors and the general public. You may run into resistance concerning your self-healing practices. This resistance may come from your closest family members and friends, your oncologist, or your surgeon. The one person in your medical team who must support you is your nutritionist/dietician. If they don't know about the twelve-grams-of-carbs-a-day diet or the rainbow diet, you may be in a backward and ignorant place and need desperately to go elsewhere. If you have no other option, it may be up to you to immediately educate and involve the nutritionists in your treatment plan.

I find it easier to overcome such resistance if I have recently listened to Dr. Tom Seyfried, Dominic D'Agostino, or Dr. Kelly Turner. It is important that you believe in what you are doing. I was trained to utilize my mind creatively. As a man believes in his heart—so he is.

# CHAPTER 11

# Other Alternative Healing Modalities

Dr. Ray Sahelian, MD, has a website that covers a wide variety of alternative treatments. It is dated July 2015, so it is relatively recent and somewhat complete. He lists the sources of his statements so you can research anything in more depth. I would not say I agree with absolutely everything, but it is a great source with a ton of information in one place. Just skip around to what applies to your specific situation.[68]

One study I found of personal interest was his section on alcohol. He quotes a study showing the link between liquor and beer and the disease, but no such link was found with wine. If the study was accurate, one might extrapolate that it might be wise for most people to switch from liquor and even beer to wine. If you are fighting the disease, any drinking may be weakening your life force. However, some disease-fighting diets allow limited consumption of red wine.

Dr. Sahelian lists a variety of herbs, vitamins, supplements, diets, foods, and alternative and natural treatments to prevent, treat, or slow down the various manifestations of this disease. His lists of herbs, supplements, and vitamins are quite extensive. I recommend not trying to do everything. Pick a handful you are drawn to or whose cultural traditions or current research makes the most sense to you.

He sticks to alternative treatments he considers respectable and legitimate. I think it is a great site, but I would be remiss if I didn't point out that he does not mention that there are even more alternative and even outlawed treatments—several of which have existed since the 1930s.

---

[68] **Search Phrase: www.raysahelian.com.**

Some serious alternative treatments, which were not fraudulent quack-ery, were outlawed by the government. Some of these therapies cure some of the participants, but they don't heal all—or even most—of the patients. But some heal however a small percentage of their patients. An abundance of alternative treatment facilities exists in Mexico because they are illegal here.

It is a huge and devastating problem that many of these alternative therapies may work for an undetermined percentage of those who try them. There will be anecdotal stories of patients who have remissions and successes, but the rest of their clients have funerals. The FDA will not tolerate claims for a cure if these alternative treatments only work for a limited percentage of patients. Out of the many clinics in Mexico some are serious, some based on lunatic fringe nonsense, and some are straight-up con jobs.

In my experience with the true mouth-to-ear mystical traditions, there are always pretenders, wannabes on the outside, posers who want to be on the inside, and people who act like they have the wisdom, power, and love of the advanced initiate without doing the work and training. These folks can range from the pretenders to the mentally unbalanced. It seems that the field of alternative cures may draw very similar person-alities. You may find the lunatic fringe wherever you have alternative healings. Even worse, con men will take advantage of the desperate. Many who fight this disease become so desperate that they naturally want to believe something will work; and may be incredibly vulnerable and easy to con.

## Alternative and Ultra-Alternative/Outlawed Therapies

The FDA attempts to be vigilant in protecting the desperately ill segment of our population, and I would like to believe they have good intentions. However, our government, in its zealous effort to protect the most des-perate people in our population, might not always get it right.

Remember how O. Carl Simonton's work was attacked at first as voodoo medicine and now is standard and conventional. With the FDA, we are talking about the government, about a bureaucratic government agency—do you think they get anything right 100 percent? You don't, and neither do I. Because of this, I will list a few of the many alternative, ultra-alternative, and outlawed therapies.

The eight-part program presented in this book was designed to be used as quickly after diagnosis as possible, hopefully at an early stage. However, there are many anecdotal stories of the twelve-gram disease-starvation diet bringing people back from the doors of death to become free and clear, sometimes in an amazingly short time. If a patient with an advanced stage of the disease was already weak and desperate, they may want to look at all their options. Desperation clouds the eyes and judgment. Don't get conned.

However, people at stage 3 or 4 may want to look at all the alternative treatments and see if there is something else that makes sense to them—something else they can believe in. Some of these alternative treatments are based on alternative theories about the cause of the disease and the way to treat the disease. If you go to www.cancertutor.com, they list many alternative treatments. Some are more controversial than others. Some of them are very far off the beaten path of science and medicine.

One alternative treatment you will find at the health food store is homeopathy. In Europe, homeopathic remedies are often used by medical doctors and the general public, and they are widely used in India, according to the Huffington Post.[69]

Here, homeopathic remedies are found at the health food store and are not prescribed by medical doctors. It is an old "like cures like" idea, in an extremely diluted solution, and was developed in 1796. Some people use them and swear by them, although some American studies don't back their validity.

If you are interested, the Nobel Prize–winning discoverer of the AIDS virus, Luc Montagnier, surprised the scientific community when he expressed his belief in homeopathy.

There are many people who use homeopathic remedies and Bach flower remedies, which are an offshoot of homeopathy. Bach flower remedies have been called vibrational medicine. If you have used homeopathy or Bach flower remedies for years and believe in them, please continue. If you get the best modern medical help, are on one of the healing diets, and do the rest of my eight-part plan and want to add homeopathy or Bach

[69] Search Phrase: www.cancertutor.com, Luc Montagnier + Homeopathy.

remedies, go for it. If they have been effective for you and you believe in them, continue using them as part of your ammunition to fight this disease.

For the interested, just put in homeopathy or Bach flower remedies, get the definitions, read the histories, look at the research, and decide from there.[70]

## The Gerson Therapy

In the field of these ultra-alternative and outlawed treatments, there are names and protocols and various theories and treatments I recognize, but most I have not studied. I chose to use the Warburg effect to metabolically fight the disease with the twelve-gram disease-starvation diet because it made the most sense to me, was logical, and was based on Nobel Prize–winning science. However, the oncology community stayed with chemo and radiation instead of switching to a metabolic treatment using a diet-based modality. If elements in the oncology community could squash a Nobel Prize–based extremely logical treatment, it makes me wonder how many other similarly squashed treatments may have some validity or efficacy.

The Gerson therapy has been around a long time and has anecdotally worked for some. I read about it years ago; it is based on diet and lifestyle. My impression at the time was you paid money, lived there, and they fed you a bunch of incredibly healthy smoothies all day. I don't remember all the details from the book, but they made claims that angered the FDA. The FDA went to war with them, and they ended up in Mexico.[71]

The Gerson Therapy clinic in Mexico, which I easily found on the internet, had you and another person stay there, preferably for three weeks. They had you walk daily and gave you thirteen smoothies and five coffee enemas a day for $60,000. So, for about $2,850 a day you can be supported by a companion, get cleaned out, and be ultra-nourished.

The goals of Gerson and the goals of my program are similar in a

---

[70] Search Phrases: cancer tutor.com, www.huffingtonpost + homeopathy in Europe and India, homeopathy, homeopathic remedies for cancer, Bach flower remedies.
[71] Search Phrase: the Gerson Therapy.

couple of ways. The shared goals are to boost the immune system and raise the level of oxygen in the blood. The anecdotal evidence is that it has worked for some stage 3 and 4 people who became free and clear survivors. It has worked for some people for eighty years. However, not every patient responds in the same way. It has worked for some people, not necessarily many, or most, and certainly not all.

## Other Alternative Treatments

The previously mentioned site where I found many alternative treatments to this disease was www.cancertutor.com. In some circumstances, photon or proton therapy is an accepted conventional alternative to normal radiation. You will also find many controversial unconventional therapies explained there such as the Cellick-Budwig protocol, a high-frequency RF protocol, the use of cesium chloride, and their own dirt-cheap protocol. Again, this stuff is not embraced by the conventional medical community, and some of it is pretty far out there. What has any real therapeutic value, what is whacky or quackery, and what is a straight-up con job?

In the treatment of many diseases, the placebo effect comes into play. In scientific testing, it was consistently found that a certain number of people respond favorably to a pill or shot containing no medicine or active ingredient. There is no other explanation than the patients expect or believe they will get better. There is also the nocebo effect, where the patients' negative expectations or beliefs make them worse.[72]

With many of these alternative therapies when the patient responds favorably, it may be very hard to distinguish whether it is the treatment or the belief of the patient.

## The Baking Soda/Vitamin C Protocol

It is hard for me to see how *some* of these alternative therapies could hurt anything, and if the person doing it believes in it, it may help them. The baking soda/vitamin C protocol seems harmless, and the theory behind

[72] **Search Phrases: the placebo effect, the nocebo effect, cancertutor.com, using the placebo effect + Harvard health.**

it does not seem absurd, when used in harmony with an extremely low-carb or ketogenic diet. Many of these alternative treatments are supposed to be used in conjunction with a healthy low-carb diet. The individual success stories that come from many of these alternative therapies may be because of the recommended changes in diet and lifestyle and the beliefs and expectations of the patients.

Cancertutor.com lists so many alternative treatments I can't go into all of them and keep this book short and simple. If you are desperate, it is natural to look at anything and everything, but don't get conned. There are unethical people who will take a sick person's last dime, and I'm not talking just about that small percentage of unethical doctors. There are people who make their living conning the desperately ill. Do your research, be skeptical, and don't get conned.[73]

## Royal Rife and the High RF Cancer Cure

In looking over the ultra-alternative and outlawed therapies, I came upon the Dr. Royal Rife story. I saw a potential parallel between his work and Warburg's. However, the scientific community accepted all of Warburg's work on the difference between the metabolism of a healthy cell and a mutant cell. They respected his Nobel Prize, but the oncology community didn't take the logical next step and embrace a metabolic theory of the disease and a dietary cure by replacing glucose with ketones and starving the mutant cells. Instead, most of the medical oncology establishment put on blinders and refused to accept a metabolic theory and refused to move away from radiation and chemo toward a metabolic cure.

Dr. Rife was a brilliant scientist, respected by his peers, but when he came up with an alternative theory for the cause and treatment for this disease, he faced unexpected animosity. He died a pauper, convinced his work had been the victim of an intentional economically based conspiracy by elements of the AMA. It would be easy for some to dismiss him; except for the fact that he was an incredibly intelligent researcher with fourteen awards from the United States government and an honorary medical degree from the University of Heidelberg.

---

[73] **Search Phrase: the baking soda/vitamin c protocol to treat cancer.**

The 1944 annual report of the board of regents of the Smithsonian Institute hailed the microscope he invented, and the photos it could provide were detailed and praised. However, when he went to Johns Hopkins to show what he could do, he ran into two very powerful critics in the medical establishment who did everything they could to discredit his claims. He died destitute and embittered, believing his work was absolutely correct and that certain elements of the AMA had conspired against him. Conspiracy theorists love his story. Interest in his work was raised by the 1987 book *The Cancer Cure that Worked: 50 Years of Suppression* by Barry Lynes.

Dr. Rife claimed to have greatly improved the microscope, saying he could find the radio wave frequency that matched an organism and could light it up making what had been difficult to see become easily visible. Then he discovered that just like a trained singer can shatter a glass, a high radio frequency could be used to destroy the microbes that he believed made a cell mutant. He believed that with the right frequency, he could destroy the bad microbes, and the mutant cells could return to being normal cells. To really understand this story in more detail, there is www.rifeviedos.com, one of many sites about this controversial, highly intelligent figure.[74]

In the article *Understanding Microbe-Induced Cancers,* we see that modern science accepts that at least three forms of this disease are caused by microbes. Dr. Rife thought all the mutations were caused by or had sustaining microorganisms, and that the right HR frequencies could destroy them. His early work was accepted by his colleagues and reported in the newspapers. He did experiments in association with USC, and his work was accepted by the Smithsonian Institute; he was a highly respected scientist until he rocked the boat. He and his work were viciously attacked when he said he could damage the mutant cancer cells with radio waves.[75]

He felt that within the AMA, within certain elements of conventional medicine, there was a very real and intentional conspiracy to discredit him and his work at all cost. If he designed radio frequency machines that people could use at home, back then for a few hundred, now a few

---

[74] Search Phrases: Royal Rife, *The Cancer Cure that Worked: 50 Years of Suppression* by Barry Lynes, and www.rifeviedos.com.
[75] Search Phrase: understanding microbe-induced cancers.

thousand dollars—that could be used daily for a few minutes and would kill the disease—what effect would that have on the medical establishment's status quo? What about lost revenue?

Who's to say that over time he may not be proved more and more correct? There may have been validity in his work that powerful well-meaning doctors just assumed was wrong because it disagreed with the prevalent theory of cause and treatments. To think radical change is always greeted with an open mind, even in medicine and science, is naïve.

## Be Skeptical

Although I didn't investigate this subject until after my surgeries and I was free and clear, I am very skeptical about people selling any purported Rife devices. Even if Rife had a device that was effective if used properly, think about how easy it would be for anyone with low morals to fake. If you are interested in this subject, you must do research and find legitimate sites.

We know sound waves can help, heal, or hurt; we know a singer can break a glass. Is it really so hard to believe that specific radio frequencies could kill harmful microbes? I found reports about how conventional scientists are looking at bacteria to see if they use radio wave communication; it is possible conventional science may catch up to and verify at least some of Rife's work.[76]

I am not endorsing his machines or his theory, but I do find him and his story highly interesting. A huge problem during his life—and currently—are dishonest people making machines they claim are like his but are total shams or have no high-frequency carrier as was used in his machines. There really seems to be only one or two manufacturers who are actually reproducing his system with a high-frequency carrier. Without it, it's not really one of his types of machines. If you are drawn to this, are well off, and have a couple of thousand you can spare, do your research.

---

[76] **Search Phrase: www.rifevideos.com.**

## Desperation

The longer one remains ill, the closer to death one grows, the more desperate they may become. The desperation I experienced was in knowing that I had a golf ball-sized mass of mutant cells in my bladder and that we needed to keep all the mutant cells where they were and get rid of them before anything else happened. I was desperate for the bad cells to stay put and then be gone. Some people reading this book are at a later stage and know a far deeper desperation than I felt. If I was extremely desperate and had the money, I would be seriously considering any therapy that made logical sense to me, had been legitimately documented to work, and that I could believe in.

I hope that if you are stage 4 and just discovered the system presented here, you would switch to my diet and implement my system if you are strong enough. I have great faith in the twelve-gram disease-starvation diet and the eight-part program I suggest. It is designed to be used at the beginning, when you are healthy enough to exercise and live an active lifestyle. If you are stage 3 or 4, get medical guidance concerning diet, exercise, and the rest of my program.

Even if you are weak, the rainbow diet may be a viable alternative. Most doctors want most patients to be as active as possible. You may be able to do the complete breath in your hospital bed. I certainly did.

## Use the Power of Belief Wisely

If I was stage 4–desperate, I'd look at any alternative treatment that made sense to me, that had worked for some, and that I could believe in. If I did research, and it made sense to me, I would be open to it—even with the clear and full understanding that most doctors think most of the ultra-alternative and outlawed treatments are quackery. It is your life; if you can easily afford it, do what you feel gives you the best chance at survival. Just apply some common sense and don't get conned.

Many of the baking soda-related treatments are inexpensive and done at home. I am less suspicious of them than treatments that cost many thousands of dollars. However, Gerson works for some people. There are low-acid theories and pH theories with adherents and detractors you can find easily on the net. Royal Rife's experiments were highly effective. If you are not strong, I would encourage you to do as much of my system as possible under medical guidance. Feel free to add other things that you can easily afford and believe in strongly.

## Marijuana

Although still technically illegal from a federal viewpoint, state after state has legalized marijuana either for medicinal purposes or for both medical and recreational use.

As someone who has suffered chronic pain every day for decades, I know marijuana is always listed as one of the top five remedies for nerve pain. Only when I began fighting this disease did I realize its other incredible curative power. Study after study shows how marijuana inhibits the growth of tumors or just kills the mutant cells outright.

All I can do is ask the reader to go to the internet and check out first the more conservative sights like the ACS—they are surprisingly receptive and positive on the subject. Check out two more sites: *twenty studies that cannabis cures cancer,* and *the top 42 studies that cannabis cures cancer.* Read any detracting studies so that you see both sides. However, the antitumor effects of cannabis are getting harder and harder to deny.[77]

Depending on the source, the effects of eating cannabis last longer than inhaling it. For those who would rather inhale, vaporizing it is much healthier than smoking because there's no burning. Both ways go into the bloodstream quicker than eating it, but the effects last a shorter period of time. In my research, nobody was prescribing it as a complete cure by itself. It was used only as a part of a larger treatment plan.

No responsible source is saying, "Go to Jamaica, sit on the beach, smoke ganja all day, and you'll get well." However, Israel and a growing number of nations allow their doctors to prescribe it as part of an intelligent and compassionate treatment plan.

Unfortunately for some advanced higher-stage patients of conventional oncologists not open to alternatives—patients whose doctors

[77] **Search Phrases: cancer + marijuana, marijuana cures cancer, "twenty studies that cannabis cures cancer" and "the top 42 studies that cannabis cures cancer."**

continue to give them chemo or radiation with no statistical expectation of a cure or serious improvement—sitting on that beach may give the patient a much higher quality of life than throwing up and being bald the last few miserable weeks of their lives.

# CHAPTER 12 ‖‖‖

# Other Alternatives

Before leaving the subject of alternative healing modalities, there are some less extreme and more mainstream alternative healing modalities that may help—even if they are not expected to cure the disease. They may help in enduring chemo or radiation or otherwise help you be healthier while you fight to regain your health.

Maybe you already know someone who practices acupuncture, acupressure, traditional Chinese herbal medicine, traditional Indian Ayurvedic medicine, therapeutic massage, Do-in, or traditional native healing from North, Central, or South America or some other part of the world. As someone trained in one of these traditions, I believe that a *genuine healer* trained in one of these fields can provide great help to the body-mind-spirit of many fighting to regain a healthy state. I've experienced acupuncture, acupressure, Do-in, massage, and traditional native healing practices and believe there is value in all these traditions.

As a practitioner of the martial arts and yoga, I would be remiss if I didn't mention what is known in yoga circles as mudra yoga, in Taoism as kuji-in, and in the Japanese martial arts as kuji-kiri. The idea here is that hands and fingers can be used to manipulate the energy of the health aura, the energy that flows through the acupuncture meridians, the energy known as prana-Chi-Ki-mana. By a mindful manipulation of the fingers and hands, the practitioner is thought to be able to raise their consciousness and obtain access to certain energies. These practices can be used for meditation and healing.[78]

The readers who like martial arts movies may have seen kuji-kiri when the ninja or other martial artist sat in meditation and took his fingers through nine forms or the nine cuts. One of these is healing. This is considered so powerful by some who practice it that at least one martial arts author referred to it as the last real magic in the modern world.

I am a great believer in how much a good full-body massage can improve your physical and mental health. Dr. Rick Agel was a practicing surgeon who now practices acupuncture. He believes it is a powerful healing modality that can really help you get through chemo or radiation much more easily. I know some people who love their chiropractors and believe that it is a powerful healing modality. I am a great believer in the Native American sweat lodge.

Whatever healing modality works for you, that you believe in, that makes you healthier, as long as it harmless, is inexpensive, or you can easily afford it—and you want to add it to the eight-part plan—go for it.


## Load Your Shotgun

There is no shortage of such healing alternatives. If you want to take advantage of one or more of these—just like in choosing a doctor—do your research on the internet and by word of mouth. Investigate as much as you can. As long as you get the best modern medical help, stay on the diet, and work the rest of my eight-part program, acupuncture, massage, and traditional herbs can only help if

- you can easily afford it,
- it doesn't hurt you or others,
- you believe it will help you,
- it helps you to get through chemo or radiation,
- it makes you feel better or more energetic, and
- your doctor or other medical professionals say it can't hurt.

---

[78] **Acupuncture + fighting cancer, acupressure + fighting cancer, Ayurvedic + fighting cancer, traditional Chinese medicine + fighting cancer, traditional Native American + fighting cancer, mudra yoga + fighting cancer, kuji-kiri.**

If so, do it along with your eight-part program. I don't want to do anything to inhibit belief in any legitimate healing modality that can genuinely help. This is the fight for your life, so load your shotgun shells with the buckshot pellets of any legitimate healing modality. A few of those pellets can hit the target and kill the disease. If you get free and clear, who cares that some of the healing modalities weren't as effective as advertised? You got well.

## Use Belief Intelligently

If you are following a strict diet and working my system as much as possible, but you want to add the vitamin C-baking soda treatment, go for it. If you have a couple of grand and want to do the high-RF treatments because you believe in them, go for it. If you want to sleep each night to 528 Hz music, go for it. If it is not antagonistic to my diet and program, if it is harmless, is logical to you, you really believe in it, and you can easily afford it, go for it. When it comes to healing, the power of belief cannot be overstated. The belief needs to be in something real, something logical, and in something that has been documented to have legitimately worked for at least some people. Don't get conned.

I express the importance of belief when facing this disease based on my experience training and working as a shaman.

## A Healable Disease

One thing I learned early in my study of shamanism—while talking with other healers in what anthropologists refer to as our *craft network*—is that some illnesses, diseases, and problems respond much better to spiritual healing than others. Because of my spinal cord injury and personal situation, I kept my ear out, and in my decades of research, I never heard of a single instance in which a medically verified severed spinal cord was healed. There are always stories, and I met a yoga guru who had the scars, the calcium formations, and a fantastic story, but I said a medically verified severed spine. I never heard of a single such case that was spiritually healed, but I heard about scores of successful spiritual healings of people fighting this disease.

Healing this disease is not making the blind see or the paralyzed walk or regenerating severed limbs. This disease is one of the most susceptible to being positively influenced by diet, lifestyle change, and spiritual healing. Documented spontaneous and radical remissions happen with this disease all over this nation because they can; they are within the scope of reality. Dr. Turner's work is fact—not science fiction.

Since I was trained as a shaman and have applied my trade for decades, we must talk about going to a healer as one of the potential alternative treatments you may consider.

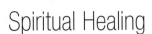

# CHAPTER 13

# Spiritual Healing

### Pranic, Psychic, Religious, and Spiritual Healing

There are many kinds of healers and a large variety of healing sessions, ceremonies, and rituals. Most organized religions currently have or have had a healing tradition as well as a mystical tradition. As someone initiated in these practices, I can break down some of the options available to one who is looking for healing outside of themselves or looking for healing to help connecting to their own higher self and the divinity within the core, center, and essence of their being.

As a mystic, I think that all healing is ultimately self-healing, that the healer helps you to get in touch with *your* higher self and the divinity within, and that the spiritual power within heals oneself. Jesus taught that the entire kingdom of heaven was within. He is far from the only great spiritual teacher to teach that all healing and all the answers are ultimately found within us—and not by looking outward. However, that doesn't mean the spiritual healer has not traditionally been needed by some to help clear the way for the internal self-healing energy. There are spiritual healers in all the cultures I know about.

### Genuine Spiritual Healing

Dr. Kelly Turner's work on spontaneous and radical remission found that most of the remissions happened over an extended period of time;

however, spontaneous remissions do happen occasionally. Healers don't exist in all cultures for no reason. Since there have been human beings, there have been healers.

Science has proved repeatedly for decades that there are people who can go into a lab and positively or negatively influence the growth of bacteria, fungi, yeast, and goiters and tumors on mice. Modern science has repeatedly proven a gifted spiritual healer can exert a quantifiable influence. In England, spiritual healers are allowed to go into hospitals to openly treat their patients. Go to an English site (www.thehealingtrust.orguk) and read "A Review of the Scientific Evidence Supporting Spiritual Healing." It reviews legitimate scientific testing that repeatedly shows a gifted healer can exert an influence.[79]

A legitimate, genuine, gifted spiritual healer can exert an influence. It might not be the overwhelming influence in that situation, but they can exert a healing influence. That doesn't necessarily mean complete remission, miraculous healing, or even any discernible healing at all, but a healing influence can be something real.

## Humans Are Multidimensional Beings

In examining the various mystical and spiritual healing traditions around the world, there are many things you will find in common. One of these commonalities is the way we divide ourselves into various aspects of a whole.

Whether the healing tradition divides a human into three aspects—like the subconscious mind, conscious mind, and the superconscious or the low, middle, and high self—the seven aspects of Vedantic Hinduism or Esoteric Section Theosophy, the nine aspects of Tibetan Hinduism, or the ten of the Kabbalists—the human being, although a single entity, is always divided into several aspects or dimensions. Every human is a multidimensional being.

String theory is up to eleven dimensions of reality. Sometimes I do blessings at weddings; before I start, I tell the couple that my belief system

---

[79] **Search Phrases: scientific proof of spiritual healing, www.thehealing-trust.orguk—evidence for spiritual healing.**

is thirty thousand to one hundred thousand years old. I tell them that someday in the future, science will get to the dimension where we work, and we shamans and mystics will be there to greet the scientists when they finally show up.

## The Multidimensional Human Being

I was taught by one of my teachers that the human being breaks down like this:

- a physical body
- an electromagnetic energy field (also called the health aura or the etheric body) that interpenetrates the physical body and extends a few inches outside of it
- an emotional aspect/emotional energy field
- a mental aspect/mental energy field
- an aspect of intuition
- a soul
- a divine spirit with a divine spark—a spark of the divine fire of the Creator

The human being has a physical body, which has a biologically based interpenetrating electromagnetic energy field that extends a few inches outside of the body. This has been variously called the *health aura* or the *etheric body* in the West. This electromagnetic energy field may relate to the life force, the Ki, Chi, prana we have been increasing through deep breathing, and also relates to the acupuncture meridians.

At the other end of this spectrum, we each are given a spark of the divine and a divine spirit. It is up to us to take that spark and make it into our own individual flame. This theory of the multidimensional human goes: physical body—etheric body—emotions—mind—intuition—soul—divine spirit/divine spark.

In the ancient mystical traditions, they would use the term *body* to mean what we refer to as an *energy field*. I would hear the human was made up of the physical body, the etheric body, the astral (emotional) body, the mental body, the intuition (which in flashes connects the mind/

awareness with the direct knowing of the spirit), the soul, and the divine spirit with a divine spark.

Here is some information for those who want to compare this system with modern psychology or Huna:

- The low self or id would be the body, the etheric body, and some of the astral.
- The middle self or ego would be some of the astral, the mental body, the intuition, and some of the soul.
- The high self, superego, or superconscious would be the highest aspects of the soul, the divine spirit, and the divine spark.

## Techniques of Spiritual Healing

Some of my teachers taught that once you accept that the human is a multidimensional being, then one of the ways to heal—in the most simplistic terms—is for the spiritual healer to clear the way for the divine spiritual healing energy of the divine spark and divine spirit of the patient to flow down through and heal:

- the soul
- the intuition
- the mind
- the emotions
- the health aura
- the physical body

Different healers in the United States and around the world use a vast variety of techniques, items, and rituals to accomplish spiritual healing. When I returned to college as an anthropology student, I had been a student of Métis Shamanism for seven years. I was an honors student in symbolic anthropology, and my professors knew about my experiences. When we would watch films from around the world, the professors would sometimes have me explain to the class what the shaman, witch doctor, or voodoo priest was doing. When it comes to healing and shamanism, there is the unique and individual, and there is the archetypical and the universal.

## A Spiritual Self-Healing Technique

Most healers want their patients to contribute actively to their own healing. When I first met Grandmother Eve, she would do her healing ceremonies, but she expected me to do my part. She utilized and smoked a Sacred Pipe in some of her healing ceremonies; other times, she would smudge everything with sage and use her eagle feathers and her healing stone. She worked on my aura and my body, but she held the firm belief that healing occurred first in the spiritual realms and then in the physical realm. She felt like she was doing her part as a shaman, but she wanted me to do my part to contribute to my own healing.

Grandmother Eve taught me one technique of spiritual self-healing that she considered extremely simple and highly effective. Agnostic and atheist readers, people like my younger brother, think this is all just imagination and delusion. However, in World War II, there was a saying that there are no atheists in a foxhole. When people face their own mortality, such firmly held beliefs may change. He is partly right in that we do use our imagination, but in a controlled and disciplined way that we believe opens us up to the infinite love of God, which is omnipresent on a higher dimension where God is love.

Our divine spark and divine spirit exist on a higher dimension and have access to—and are literally bathed in—divine love. However, that doesn't mean our soul-intuition-mind-emotions-body have automatic access to this energy.

## The Spiritual Reality of Divine Love

In the mystical worldview, everything vibrates naturally. There are extremely high and extremely low frequencies—and everything in between. The lower frequencies of the earth plane and id—the frequencies of your instincts, carnal desires and emotions, selfish thoughts, feelings, possessive loves, angers, and hatreds—are in no way the same vibe or frequency as that of divine love.

One must quiet the mind and train the imagination to reach inward and upward at the same time, to reach that level of divine love—of unconditional love—where God is love. This energy, according to the mystical tradition, can heal almost anything. The way you reach in and up, the way you reach the God is love level, is through the intention to commune with your own divine spirit and spark.

Before going into Grandmother Eve's technique, Ruth Stillman, an Esoteric Section-trained Theosophist used to lead a short meditation that can make Grandmother Eve's technique much more effective.

## Ruth's Powerful Meditation

Ruth's meditation goes like this:

First, you must consciously relax your body, especially the muscles of the neck and shoulders, of the face, around the eyes, and of the scalp. Relax your body completely, close your eyes, and breathe deeply several times. Mentally go through your body from head to feet or vice versa and make sure all the major muscle groups, that all the voluntary muscles, are relaxed.

When you are completely relaxed, begin a series of statements that are used in this meditation to carry your consciousness up through your multidimensional being, from your body to your divine spark.

With your eyes closed, sitting up straight but completely relaxed, you say (out loud, in a whisper, or internally) and think and feel the first statement, and then take a deep breath, and say and think and feel the next statement, etc. If you need to take more than one breath at a level, before moving up, let your intuition guide you.

## Ruth Stillman's Meditation

Take a deep breath as you say, feel, and think the following:

- I have a body, but I am not just my body.
- I have an etheric body, but I am not just my etheric body.
- I have emotions, but I am not just my emotions.
- I have a mind, but I am not just my mind.
- I have intuition, but I am more than my intuition.
- I have a soul, but I am more than my soul.
- I am a divine immortal spirit with a spark of the divine eternal flame (a spark of the all-powerful, infinite, and all-loving God).

You rest here in the knowledge of and identification with your own divine immortal spirit and divine spark.

After what you feel is the appropriate time, come back down through each level to return to your body—in the knowledge that you are a created divine immortal spirit.


## Eve's Self-Healing Technique

Immediately after Ruth's meditation is an ideal time to do Grandmother Eve's spiritual self-healing technique. The theory used here is that the etheric, astral, mental, and spiritual worlds are plastic and moldable, according to the exercise of controlled thought and will. Grandmother Eve used the symbol of the circle, which she felt the Indians used extensively and was also a universal symbol and spiritual tool, widely used around the world.

To begin, she would use her imagination or hand (first two fingers pointing, back two fingers forming circle with thumb) and draw and form a small circle of white light above her head in her imagination, beginning in the north and moving clockwise above her head to the east, then south, then west, then back to north. Then she would point-draw-imagine a larger similar clockwise circle of white light on the floor/ ground around her.

Then she would imagine or call forth a circular column of divine spiritual white light, (known in different traditions as the divine white light, the Christ light, or the limitless light) coming down to the first circle and spreading to the larger circle on the floor, forming a cone of white light. It is as though by using the symbol of the circle, Eve had called or invoked a column of white light coming down from above. She would imagine it forming hundreds of feet above her head, pouring down as a circular column into the circle above her, filling the cone with the divine love of God.

She would imagine the omnipresent dimension of reality where God is love, the realm where her divine spark and spirit reside, and she would use her imagination to call down, bring down the divine white light—called in some of the mystical traditions the Christ light—by whatever tradition known as the divine love of God—to make its healing way down.

Down from the dimension of divine spirit, in a circular column of white light, comes the healing white light of divinity—down into and through the dimensions, planes, levels—of the soul, the intuition, the mind, the emotions, the health aura, down to the physical body.

The self-healer can take their passive hand and hold it, very relaxed, palm up. In the imagination, the self-healer can allow this bright white light to pour like a circular spotlight into the passive hand and out of the palm of the active hand like a spotlight of luminous healing energy. The self-healer can direct the energy from above the head (the divine lotus or crown chakra) down through the aura/body to a central point below the feet (called by some the earth star).

This drawing down of the spiritual energy from above the head to below the feet as directed by the motion of the palm can be repeated, very slowly, pouring the white light out of the active hand like an intense spotlight of spiritual energy going down the middle of the body, then going down each side, filling the body with divine white light.

The white light, as it goes in one palm and comes out the other, is as a bright healing spotlight of divine white light energy. It can be directed at specific body parts in need of healing. You can fill any area or organ with the white light, and once you have, you will usually conclude the session with the downward flowing palm. You want the overall energy to be flowing freely through your energy bodies/meridians, from above your head to below your feet, and you want your energy flowing freely.

Another esoteric version of this healing technique has the divine white light originating from the center or heart of the (spiritual) sun, pouring forth to the atmosphere of the earth, coming down as a column of white light to the top circle, forming and filling the cone of white light, and from the bottom of the cone, it travels as a column of white light going down into the center of the earth our mother, to heal her at the same time we heal ourselves. In Native American and other traditions, the earth is considered a living being, and because of all the damage done by humans, it is in need of healing as well.[80]

When one practices this spiritual self-healing technique, it is not unusual to have confirming sensations in the receiving and pouring hand. To me, it feels like a gentle breeze is blowing in and out around my fingers and palms. Others feel warmth, tingling, or a pouring sensation. Eve said some may not have such confirmatory sensations at first, but that didn't mean the technique wasn't working.

Once Grandmother Eve told me that the eagle feathers and healing stones used by shamans did have a power unique to themselves, which might be intensified through the repeated usage of such spiritual healing tools. However, she said that the exact same results could be obtained through the practice of this technique without the use of healing tools or complex rituals. She said that such spiritual tools like the feathers and healing stone were used primarily to increase the belief of the patient and were not necessary for healing to occur. She believed firmly in the power and efficacy of this self-healing technique.

If you believe at some level or dimension there is a reality where God is love, why not use the mental tools available to you to become open to and receive the healing energy of divine love?

## Purification and Cleansing

In many cultures before and after doing any such healing technique or ritual, there may be a symbolic and physical cleansing performed by the healer. This is a purification, washing away, or casting off any possible negative energy. This is often done with sage or incense or by washing one's hands.

In many healing ceremonies or rituals around the world, there is an act of ceremonial purification before and cleansing after. This may be a combination of physical actions with symbolic intentions. For indigenous

---

[80] **Search Phrase: healing the earth mother.**

Americans, this act before and after may involve smudging—the use of the smoke of burning sage like many institutional religions use incense. The individual will take a handful of smoke and then bring it down from above the head to purify the front, back, and both sides.

Depending on the views of the healer and patient in healing rituals or sessions, the healer (or self-healer) may believe they are bringing in positive higher-frequency spiritual healing energy and replacing the lower-frequency negative unhealthy disease energy. Shamans around the world can be seen taking the negative energy out of the aura/body and replacing it with positive energy. In many traditions, it is cast down into the earth for the earth to take and purify.

In the same way that garbage is cast into the compost heap and becomes nutritious fertilizer for your yard, the shaman will take the negative energy and wash it or shake it off into the earth. What has been garbage (disease energy) to the patient is symbolically given to Mother Earth who takes it like compost to bless and nurture the earth. Many healers will do some obvious symbolic purification beforehand. I have seen some preparations that were as simple as rubbing one's hands together. However, almost all healers I know do some form of purification before and cleansing after such healing techniques.

Unless I'm outside where I would symbolically shake my fingers in a casting-off motion toward the earth, I just go to the sink and wash my hands with the intention of washing away any and all unhealthy energy, guilt, sin, or negative energy I have come into contact with.

As with most of this, find what works for you. Depending on your spiritual traditions, many of you may already have altars for your spiritual practice. You may already have your own forms of purification and cleansing you use before and after your prayers.

Pranic Healing

Other forms of healing may claim the title "spiritual," but they are not genuine spiritual healing. Pranic healing is something I experienced once decades ago, and I will never forget the experience. Grandmother Eve invited me to come and stay for a while and introduced me to Grandfather Raymond. He granted me the honor of conducting a four-day healing sweat for me, aimed at getting me back on my feet and curing my paralysis. It is a long story; those interested can find my book *The Shaman between Worlds* by R. E. Day, Jr. on Amazon.com.[81]

The four-day healing sweat was a grueling, wonderful, incredible, life-changing event. On the fourth and final day, it took all my reserves of energy to crawl out of the Northern Paiute sweat lodge and transfer from the ground up into my wheelchair. That action took every last bit of energy I had left, and I slumped down in the chair, completely spent, thoroughly exhausted.

Grandmother Eve came up from behind me and put one hand on either shoulder. I could hear her taking deep long breaths, and she began to literally breathe life and energy into me. After she did her breathing technique for a short time, I sat up, got my shoulders back, and began to function again. When she took her hands off my shoulders, we headed into the community room for the ceremonial meal.

Pranic healing is the building up and transferring of prana, life force, Ki, or Chi by an act of breath and will. I have read about it in the lore of Hatha yoga and pranayama breath control, but that was the only time I ever experienced it. This is not spiritual healing; it is the temporary energizing of another person through a buildup and transfer of prana.

Most Western doctors and scientists don't believe this is even possible. Most don't believe in the concept of prana or a transferable, directed spiritual healing energy. I don't expect atheist or agnostic readers to buy into all of this. I don't believe all of my readers' minds will be open to accepting spiritual healing as a powerful reality. What I experienced in the Northern Paiute sweat lodge changed my mind forever on that score. For readers who can't accept that reality, don't go to a healer. I'm not telling anyone to seek a healer at all; if you are so inclined, just be intelligent about it and try to find someone who is sincere and gifted. Genuine spiritual healers are not about the money. Con men are about the money. Do not get taken.

---

[81] **Search Phrase:** *The Shaman between Worlds* **by R. E. Day, Jr. available on Amazon.com.**

## Psychic Healing

Psychic healing is also not spiritual healing. A wide variety of religious and individual practices might be considered psychic healing. This is where healers either knowingly or subconsciously attempt to use their emotions or their minds to will the person to be healed. Often, if successful at all, the patient temporarily feels better, but there is no lasting improvement. Some of the healing practices used currently in *some* Christian churches are completely driven by emotion and are not real spiritual healing, and the uplifting effects are often temporary.

## Religious and Spiritual Healing

The Christian religion always had spiritual healing as an element. In fact, much of Jesus's reputation was built on his miracles and healing. Jesus said that even greater things his followers would do; many saints were healers and many saints are called on for healing. If you are Catholic, you are familiar with the healing saints and the healing power of Holy Communion.

If you are Protestant, you are familiar with Communion and the gifts or powers of the Holy Spirit—one of which is healing. I was taught by some of my teachers that a true spiritual healer would never charge money, but that it was all right in some cases to accept donations. However, we live in one of the most materialistic cultures in human history, and many people only respect and have high expectations for what they pay for, and the more they pay, the more they expect. I am conflicted and see both sides.

Like the other alternative therapies, religious healing doesn't work for everyone. I know a couple of good folks who are friends of my brother and the husband is fighting a different but progressively debilitating disease. They have gone in search of healing. They paid one lady $5,000 for healing sessions and saw no improvement. They went to an internationally famous healer in Brazil, John of God, and saw no improvement. Then they went to Panama for experimental stem cell therapy.

Unfortunately, the disease continues. They spent many, many thousands of dollars for dubious results. Sadly, this is way too common.

Although healing might be part of the human potential, most people aren't gifted spiritual healers—and there is a con man around every corner. Even if you go to a genuinely gifted spiritual healer, there is no guarantee that you will be healed or see any improvement. In the same way we have musical geniuses, mathematical geniuses, and incredibly gifted athletes, we have gifted healers, powerful shaman, Protestants with the gift of healing, and Catholic healers who became saints. Not many people in my experience are like Grandfather Raymond or Grandmother Eve. At the same time, you can go anywhere and find talented musicians. You should be able to find a regionally gifted healer in whatever tradition or culture you belong to. If you are going to benefit from spiritual healing, you shouldn't have to travel too far or spend too much money to find someone.

One of my teachers taught that if a patient was in need of and open to spiritual healing, they would be able to find a healer and the healing energy would flow down. In the seventies, they used phrases conveying a healer's job was to *channel the energy,* be an *open channel*, or be an *open vessel* through which the divine *God is love* healing energy would flow. This teacher insisted if they were ready and looking and it was meant to be, they would find someone who could be that open channel. The healing energy would flow through the healer to the patient.

An intelligent person must contrast that ideal to all the people like my brother's friends who spent thousands of dollars in absolute desperation and got nothing. This is quite a contrast. How spiritual can anyone be who wants a lot of money for a healing ceremony?

If you want to experience effective spiritual healing, I would hope you wouldn't have to travel too far to find a gifted healer in your cultural milieu. My heritage is Scots-Irish, Irish, Scottish, English, Cherokee, and Creek, but I ended up studying under a Canadian-born Métis Shaman and a Northern Paiute shaman. I was raised a Southern Baptist but found my spiritual home at a Northern Paiute sweat lodge run by a traditional shaman, healer, and medicine man who was also a Christian.

Christians often say the Lord works or moves in mysterious ways. I would say life happens in mysterious ways for everybody. I can't say what you should do or go through on your self-healing journey, but I know Grandfather Raymond and Grandmother Eve were not healers for money; it was their calling and not their profession.

## Psychic Healing and Spiritual Aid

Psychic healing can be the attempt by one individual to use the psyche to will you to better health, or it can be one person directing the heightened frenzied emotions of many. Generally speaking, psychic healing does not bring about genuine long-term healing unless the healing ceremony or ritual experience facilitates real changes in the personality of the individual, which brings about genuine spiritual healing.

Most cultures have spiritual aid available to help you in your self-healing journey. That aid may come in the office of angels and archangels for the Judeo-Christian or as animal spirits, spirit powers, totem spirits, and grandfather spirits for the indigenous peoples of the Americas.

The definition of shaman is *master of spirits*. My book *The Shaman between Worlds* covers this subject in more detail. In many indigenous cultures, it is the norm for a person to have an animal spirit, a clan or totem spirit, or a spirit guardian. In many Christian cultures, a guardian angel or patron saint may be expected to help you when you reach out. In some examples their very existence or reason for being in your spiritual worldview is to provide you with spiritual help.

## Receiving Healing

If you grew up in such a culture and believed in your guardian angel, patron saint, guardian spirit, animal spirit, or totem animal spirit, but fell away from such beliefs as an adult, you could reach out for help. Ask your guardian angel or animal spirit to clear the path for the power of your divine spirit to heal you, and as you do, always present an energized picture of yourself healed in the present tense.

If you grew up in or converted into a culture with such belief systems and have never lost faith, you have probably been asking for such help all along. Your guardian angel, guardian spirit, or revered ancestor can be part of your spiritual ammunition with which to fight. As long as you are getting the best of modern medicine, strictly adhering to one of the diets, and working my eight-part plan, you should take advantage of all the spiritual help available to you within your cultural worldview and belief system.

Always remember to pray while presenting a picture of health in the present tense. From the middle self, see yourself free and clear, get your low self to energize that image, and present it to your guardian angel, patron saint, clan totem, personal animal spirit, or any other appropriate spiritual ally.

In whatever manner you may pray and seek spiritual aid, whether it is to your own higher self, Jesus, some angel or archangel, some other aspect of divinity from any of the world's religions, or some other spiritual intermediary—whatever you believe in—always give an energized picture of yourself healthy and well, free and clear, and in the present tense.

Invite the healing white light of whatever religion you believe in; invite the Christ light, or the love of God the Father, or the love of the divine mother to bless and heal you. Invite the divine healing power inherent within your divine spark and divine spirit to pour down, through your soul, intuition, mind, emotions, etheric body, and physical body—to bless you and heal you.

In whatever manner, it may occur—whether your remission is spontaneous, is radical over time, or however you can make it happen—work to be free and clear, have faith and belief, and work in every way you can to win the big fight. You should do this intelligently. Load your shotgun carefully and wisely. Do not give in to the desperation for healing and get conned out of thousands of dollars. True healers are not in it for the money.

# CHAPTER 14

# Those in Need of Healing—Beware

We haven't covered the whole field of chakras, energy work, Reiki, or therapeutic hypnosis, and there is an absolute ton of information available about whatever might interest you. Much of such information is totally legit. There is also a ton of garbage right next to something legitimate. You must investigate, use your powers of discernment and critical thinking, and don't get conned.

When it comes to people who claim to be healers, many are fakes and liars. There are a whole lot of talkers—some are full of BS, some are mentally ill, and some are con men who will take you for a rube—and every dollar you have—no matter how sick you are. It is easy to pretend to be spiritual. The lunatic fringe can show up in healing circles. Listen to your intuition, what draws your highest instincts, and not what pulls at your lowest. Do research online and by word of mouth.

A real healer isn't doing it for money. I never took money for healing, although once under extreme pressure from my respected teacher Ruth Stillman, I accepted a small fee under the guise of gas money. I must also admit to accepting small appreciation presents after someone got well such as a small rug or personal artwork, but there was never an expectation for such gifts. I felt it would have been rude to refuse them.

I also understand the very strong suspicion in society that anything free is without worth—that what is free has no real value. The prevalence of such a belief is reason enough for some healers to charge money and may be necessary in some places. Certainly, a hypnotherapist, chiropractor, massage therapist, or any such professional will and should charge their normal professional rate.

There are a wide variety of books on self-healing, self-improvement, New Age, yoga, Qi Gong, self-discovery, muscle testing, pendulums, and many other such related topics. I cannot possibly cover everything. If you are interested in something and have an intuitive feeling it can help you, you can find information about it on the net. Get local and start practicing whatever interests you and will make you healthier. Be discerning, use your intellect and your intuition, and don't get conned. There is a con man or woman around every corner who will look you in the eyes and lie their heads off.

Real yoga is good, real Qi Gong is good, and ethical guided relaxation and meditation can be good. Do whatever you are healthy enough to do if it is good for you and can't hurt you.

Always do research, read reviews, ask questions, and ask your friends. Don't get conned. You are being warned again and again because this field is fraught with charlatans and con men. If you are not discerning, you will be taken advantage of because you are desperate—and the desperate make easy prey.

You have been provided here with an effective and workable eight-part plan to boost your immune system and activate your self-healing mechanisms. I would like to think that it is enough all by itself, but I don't believe in restricting thought or belief systems.

You can't do everything out there. Always limit your healing supplements, exercise, alternative healing modalities, and the number of people on your prayer lists to a small, manageable, and efficient number. Focus on self-healing. You dig a well deeply in one place to reach the water of life—not with a hundred scattered shallow holes.

I am a great believer in the healing effects of a good massage, but don't ever do anything you feel might move mutant cells around. If your intuition tells you not to do something, don't do it.

There are many well-meaning and legitimate alternative and supplemental treatments and therapies. Your only constraints may be logistics, finances, time, or energy—just make sure you have applied common sense, done thorough research, and are confident you are not being conned. Once you have done your research, then do what genuinely makes you feel better and become healthier.

Whatever your belief system may be, use it to become better and healthier. In my personal worldview, that means I hope you are open to the divine within the core, center, and essence of your being.

Take Charge!

If you are a patient of a conventional oncologist who is not open to healing diets, integrative oncology, or alternative treatments—and for whatever reason you feel she or he is your best or only option—it is up to you to take charge of your lifestyle changes and alternate treatments. You are in charge of your body and your treatments, and you must decide what you need from the conventional oncologists' three weapons—surgery, chemo, or radiation—and what you want or don't want from the alternative world.

I was lucky. Although my urological surgeon wasn't holistic, he treated every individual as a unique person and didn't blindly follow protocols written decades earlier. Dr. Paul Young thought I was free and clear after the two surgeries and didn't need chemo or radiation. They were cool with a wait-and-watch approach—and so was I.

I've been free and clear for over five years. Some people may think I'm rushing the clock, that I haven't been free and clear long enough to write this book. I'm simply writing the book I wish I'd been handed that first day when my life changed.

I'm not saying everyone who tries this eight-part program will get well. They won't. That would not be in harmony with nature. A certain percentage of people who get this disease will pass away. I believe with all my heart that when large numbers of patients are compared, people who follow this plan will do much, much better statistically than patients who continue to eat a sugar-rich, normal American diet, people who do not exercise, breathe deeply, visualize, use affirmation, meditate, or pray. People who passively go through conventional treatment with a normal fast-food American diet, without herbs, vitamins, supplements, and blindly follow whatever the first doctor says will not do as well as people on my eight-part plan.

People using this eight-part plan will be doing everything they can to live clean and jack their immune systems into overdrive. These other people are leaving it up to the scalpel, radiation, or chemotherapy. I give my people something more to believe in than just a poison.

Although I'm no longer on the strict ketogenic diet I was on while fighting the disease, I continue to try to eat clean, exercise, meditate, pray, ride my motorcycle, and live my life. As a third-degree black belt in American Kenpo Karate, I run a dojo in the Atlanta suburbs.

Whenever I can, I tell people about the metabolic way to fight this disease, and the body-mind-spirit approach to winning this, the biggest fight of your life. I'm telling everybody I can.

# CONCLUSION

I have written for you the book I wish I had been handed that first day of my diagnosis. This system is what made sense to me and seems to have worked well for me. I can only wait expectantly for the results of my readers who aggressively follow this program—with a strong will to be free and clear. I will gladly compare the results of thousands of my eight-part plan people against thousands of similar patients treated conventionally with no change in lifestyle or diet. Our results will crush theirs.

You have read the book and understand our system:

- Get the best in modern medicine, take control, and decide what you want to do.
- Change your diet to aggressively starve or fight the disease.
- Visualize yourself healthy, free, and clear.
- Use positive affirmations.
- Do cardiovascular exercises and weight training.
- Do a deep breathing stretching exercise like yoga, Tai Chi, or Qi Gong.
- Do a complete breath session three times daily.
- Meditate to alleviate stress, tension, and fear.
- Pray for others and then yourself.
- Raise your vibes—bathe every day and sing or chant in the tub— use sound creatively to heal yourself—watch comedies, (adults make love), have fun, observe nature, and do whatever you can to raise your vibes.

By eating clean food, drinking pure water, and avoiding as many toxins as possible, you can allow your immune system to concentrate on defeating the disease. Using herbs, vitamins, and supplements, you can jack your immune system into overdrive. By getting good nutrition, the right kind and amount of exercise, adequate sleep, and regular deep breathing, you are reinforcing your immune system and bringing it to optimum efficiency so it can defeat this terrible disease—and you can be free and clear.

You have been taught to use the vast power of your conscious mind/ego/middle self, your subconscious mind/id/lower self, and your superconscious mind/superego/higher self to activate your self-healing mechanisms by using visualizations, affirmations, meditation, and prayer. You can do all this. It will be a full-time job. It is probably best done under the guidance of an integrative oncologist, but that is a luxury I did not have—and probably most of you will not have.


Things Keep Getting Better!

I was the primary and only caretaker of my ninety-one-year-old father when I was diagnosed. I had to cook and feed and keep him clothed while I fought the battle. At the beginning, while I was trying to figure out my diet, I often felt like I was fighting all by myself. However, I was guided by two very knowledgeable and kind people at my health food store, and I had the one book (*Fight Cancer with a Ketogenic Diet*) and the charts I used religiously to keep my diet right at the twelve grams of carb target. That was pretty much it for nutrition. I just winged it and did the best I could. Just five years later, it is so much easier to learn about these things. There is an abundance of new information on the net. Watching people in our culture work to defeat this disease in this way is a dynamic and wonderful thing to observe.

Apart from my struggles in trying to figure out my diet, I had great family and friend support. My brother Andy flew with me on the disastrous trip to Houston, and my brother Stephen drove me to Mayo until I was free and clear and strong enough to drive myself. My sister, Marguerite; my friends Tom and Deb, Laura, Christina, and Karen; my cousins Emmel and Derrell; and all my friends and family were a constant source of support. Everyone in my family-and-friend network was strong and unwavering, and I appreciated them all. Tom gave this manuscript a much-needed preliminary editing, which I greatly appreciate.

In the beginning, when it came to diet and how to fight this disease—at home, taking care of my aging father—I sometimes felt like I was alone in the dark. I felt that way off and on during my journey. It doesn't matter how positive we try to remain; every one of us will have those alone-in-the-dark moments. At those times, we must remind ourselves that we are fighting. We are fighting hard, fighting well, and doing our part. Those alone-in-the-dark moments will pass. We all have them. It's another freebie that comes along with the diagnosis.

Just five years later, things are so different now. There are new worlds of information to guide you, help you, and aid you. This way of fighting the disease is growing in popularity very rapidly, and this groundswell is becoming increasingly difficult for the conventional modern medical community to ignore. The fact that integrative oncology exists is proof of that.

However unconsciously or consciously motivated by profits it may be, ignorance within the medical community about cancer as a metabolic disease, the Warburg Effect, and the twelve-grams-of-carbs-disease-starvation diet must come to an end. The medical schools must teach the Warburg effect and teach that cancer is a metabolic disease that should be treated metabolically. Oncologists must embrace the Warburg effect, and hospitals must embrace the Warburg effect, even if it costs them all millions of dollars.

They must do this because these institutions exist to heal people; when faced with the reality of our successes, a time will come when a tipping point is reached and they can no longer ethically ignore us. They will have no choice but to embrace it, much as O. Carl Simonton's work was initially fiercely fought and later embraced.

The dieticians, nutritionists, holistic doctors, and integrative oncologists must lead the fight against this suppression. In the same way O. Carl Simonton was ridiculed by his peers, there will be haters who will attack my ideas about self-healing and this book.

When large numbers of people use these techniques aggressively—as the work of Dr. Kelly Tuner shows—when motivated self-healers follow the strategies and practices presented in this book, they will be statistically much more successful than the passive patients who do whatever their first doctor tells them to do. We will be significantly more successful than people who don't exercise and keep eating sugar-rich diets.

If you review the information on the internet about fighting the disease this way—the Seyfried, D'Agostino, and Turner YouTube videos and all the instructional YouTube videos on diet and exercise—you will find many commonalities. Don't be overwhelmed by the variety of things available. Trust your intuition. Find what you are drawn to, what you like doing, and what is easy or natural for you to do in the beginning. Don't try to do everything at once. Take things step by step and day by day.

Once people start a small, disciplined practice, it seems to grow on its own accord. It snowballs. Once you start, you just keep habitually doing it, adding bits here and there. Start dieting, exercising, and working the program in small steps if necessary. Let your own personal self-healing system grow organically. Forgive yourself, love yourself, and don't guilt-trip yourself if you can't do everything every day. Just do the best you can.

This is your life. Trust your intuition—and do what is truly best for you. Find purpose and meaning in this struggle and in the other aspects of your life as well. Life is sacred, and your life is sacred, and unless your intuition tells you your time on this earth plane is up, it is your sacred duty to fight for your life with all you have.

I have given you my eight-part plan with many ways to supercharge your immune system and activate your inherent self-healing mechanisms. You have been presented with a variety of ammunition to load into your self-healing shotgun to shoot at the disease. Scientifically speaking, not all the ammunition you've loaded into your shotgun shells may effectively strike the target. However, it may only take a few of the pellets hitting the target to kill the disease. Although we may discover at some future time that it is the combination of all the ammunition you loaded that helps those fatal pellets to find their mark and kill the disease.

Not everyone who uses this book will be healed. This disease is one mechanism nature uses when your time on this planet is up. If your time is up, may you go gracefully at home surrounded by those you love—or maybe on that beach in Jamaica.

But if your time on this planet is not up, if you have reasons to live—people to take care of, plans to see through, things you must do, or you hear the calling to live a more spiritual life—then you must fight like a tiger. Every day, fight and fight. Fight with a smile and a positive state of mind. With the right diet, with your body, mind, and spirit, fight and fight. With visualization, positive affirmation, meditation, prayer, and raising your vibes, fight and fight against this disease until you win.

I hope, wish, and pray you hear the words "free and clear" and hear them soon. I know your joy will be indescribable.

# ENDNOTES

Chapter 1: The Diagnosis and the Fight

Search Phrase: miraculous cures for cancer + injecting disease
Search Phrase: mystical tradition

Chapter 2: It Is Your Fight—and No One Else's

Search Phrases: everything vibrates, everything has frequency, all natural objects have a frequency
Search Phrase: integrative oncology, superconscious
Search Phrases: Norman Cousins, Laughter Therapy, and *Anatomy of an Illness*
Search Phrases: your diagnosis (your specific type and stage of cancer) + chemotherapy, your diagnosis + radiation, your diagnosis + surgery, your diagnosis + holistic therapies.
Search Phrases: your doctor's name + reviews, your doctor's practice + reviews
Search Phrases: sugar + cancer, FDG PET Scan + glucose, diets that fight cancer, Diets that defeat cancer, Diets that starve cancer; On YouTube: #TalkingKeto: Professor Tom Seyfried, and Starving Cancer: Dominic D'Agostino at TEDx

Chapter 3: Diets That Fight the Disease

Search phrases: Nobel Prize + Otto Warburg, the rainbow diet to fight cancer, the 12 grams of carbs a day diet to starve cancer

Search Phrases: Starving Cancer: Dominic D'Agostino at TEDx at Tampa Bay, #TalkingKeto: Professor Tom Seyfried
Search Phrase: the ketogenic diet to starve cancer
Internet Sites on the subject:
*KetoDietResource.com* and *KetoNutrition.org*
Books on the subject:
*Cancer as a Metabolic Disease* by Thomas Seyfried
*The Cantin Ketogenic Diet* by Elaine Cantin (dairy-free)
*Fight Cancer with a Ketogenic* Diet by Ellen Davis
Search Phrase: Is cancer a metabolic disease?
Search Phrases: herbs to fight + your diagnosis, vitamins to fight + your diagnosis, supplements to fight + your diagnosis
Search Phrase: the rainbow *Diet* to beat cancer
Search Phrase: low carb bread, cloud bread

Chapter 4: Eat, Drink, Breathe Clean

Search Phrase: O. Carl Simonton, boosting your immune system
Search Phrase: the complete breath
Search Phrases: on YouTube: Dr. Pierce + the complete breath
Search Phrase: oxygen + best places for deep breathing, best places for clean air, how is oxygen produced?
Search Phrase: www.raysahelian.com (scroll down and click on cancer)
Search Phrases: purifying water, GE water filter pitcher

Chapter 5: Using Your Mind Positively

Search Phrases: environmental dangers in the home, environmental dangers in the workplace
Search Phrase: percent of immune system in gut
Search Phrase: immune system + kills cancer cells

Chapter 6: Visualization and Affirmation

Search Phrase: visualization + fighting cancer
Search Phrase: affirmation + defeating cancer

Search Phrase: positive attitude + fighting cancer
Search Phrases: yoga, Qi Gong, Medical Qi Gong, Tai Chi, Michio Kushi

Chapter 7: Causation, Your Spiritual Beliefs, and the "Why Me?" Question

Search Phrase: Evelyn Eaton
Search Phrases: dangers of radio alarm clocks, danger + electromagnetic pollution, danger + EMF, EMR
Search Phrases: chronic depression + higher cancer risk, chronic depression + weakened immunity, Dr. Norman Shealy
Search Phrases: O. Carl Simonton, simontoncenter.com, and his books *Getting Well Again, The Healing Journey*
Search Phrase: Whole Armor of God
Search Phrases: St. Augustine, St. Jerome, and Origen (founding fathers of the early church and believers in reincarnation)
Search Phrases: mystical tradition + reincarnation, Justinian outlawed reincarnation
Search Phrases: Duke + reincarnation + Rhine; U of VA med school + reincarnation
Search Phrase: things to avoid + prevent cancer

Chapter 8: Prayer and Meditation Prayer

Search Phrase: the healing power of prayer
Search Phrase: Christine Sheldon—*How to Change Your Frequency to Change your Life*
Search Phrases: Huna, Max Freedom Long, healing with Huna
Search Phrases: meditation, the benefits of meditation
Search Phrases: Life force, prana, Qi or Chi, Ki, Mana; yoga, Tai Chi, Qi Gong, Do-in; Medical Qi Gong, on YouTube *Healing and Cancer— Qi Gong*
Search Phrases: healing sounds
Search Phrases: Dr. Len Horowitz, 528 hertz, and the Solfeggio and Fibonacci sequences
Search Phrases: science of Cymatics, sound as a weapon

Search Phrases: Dr. Masaru Emoto, books by Masaru Emoto
Search Phrases: the healing power of words, kotodama
Search Phrase: chanting the name of God
Search Phrase on YouTube: How to chant aum, Healing Chants, Nam-myoho-renge-kyo
Search Phrases: How to chant aum, aum, Om, Om mani padme hum

Chapter 9: Exercising—Western and Eastern

Search Phrases: How much exercise should a cancer patient get each week, Cancer and activity, Cancer and exercise
Search Phrase: the importance of cancer support groups
Search Phrase: exercise programs + fighting cancer
Search Phrases: Qi Gong + healing cancer, Dragon and Tiger Medical Qi Gong, yoga + healing cancer, Medical Qi Gong
Search Phrase: healing and cancer—Qi Gong
Search Phrase: fighting cancer + raising children, fighting cancer + while working, oncology social workers

Chapter 10: Radical Remission

Search Phrase: Dr. Kelly Turner + radical remission
Search Phrases: Dr. Kelly A. Turner's book *Radical Remission: Surviving Cancer against All Odds*, and her online course www.radicalremission.com

Chapter 11: Other Alternative Healing Modalities

Search Phrase: www.raysahelian.com
Search Phrase: Luc Montagnier + Homeopathy
Search Phrases: cancer tutor.com, www.huffingtonpost + homeopathy in Europe and India, homeopathy, homeopathic remedies for cancer, Bach flower remedies
Search Phrase: the Gerson Therapy
Search Phrases: the placebo effect, the nocebo effect, cancertutor.com, using the placebo effect + Harvard health
Search Phrase: the baking soda/vitamin c protocol to treat cancer

Search Phrases: Royal Rife, and the book *the Cancer Cure that Worked—50 Years of Suppression* by Barry Lynes.
Search Phrase: *understanding microbe induced cancers*
Search Phrase: www.rifevideos.com
Search Phrases: cancer + marijuana, marijuana cures cancer

Chapter 12: Other Alternatives

Search Phrases: acupuncture + fighting cancer, acupressure + fighting cancer, Ayurvedic + fighting cancer, traditional Chinese medicine + fighting cancer, traditional Native American + fighting cancer, mudra yoga + fighting cancer, kuji-kiri

Chapter 13: Spiritual Healing

Search Phrases: scientific proof of spiritual healing, www.thehealingtrust.orguk—evidence for spiritual healing
Search Phrase: *The Shaman between Worlds* by R. E. Day, Jr. on Amazon.com.

Made in the USA
Columbia, SC
13 June 2022

61672022R00098